Healing the Healer

The Addicted Physician

DANIEL H. ANGRES, M.D.

G. DOUGLAS TALBOTT, M.D.

KATHY BETTINARDI-ANGRES, M.S., R.N.

First Paperback Printing, 2002

Copyright © 2012, Daniel H. Angres, G. Douglas Talbott, Kathy Bettinardi-Angres.

Library of Congress Cataloging-in-Publication Data

Angres, Daniel H.
Healing the healer : the addicted physician / Daniel H. Angres, G. Douglas Talbott, Kathy Bettinardi-Angres.
P- cm.
Includes bibliographical references and indexes.
ISBN 1-887841-15-6
1. Physicians — Substance use. 2. Physicians — Drug use.
3. Substance abuse — Patients. 4. Addicts. I. Talbott, G. Douglas
(George Douglas), 1924– II. Bettinardi-Angres, Kathy.
In. Title.
[DNLM: 1. Substance-Related Disorders — therapy. 2. Physician
Impairment_ WM 270 A593h 1998]
RC564.5.M45 IN PROCESS
362.29′088′61 — c1c21
DNLM/DLC
for Library of Congress 98-15857 CIP

ISBN: 1468150677
ISBN 13: 9781468150674

Printed by CreateSpace

For the doctors, nurses, dentists, pharmacists,
and other health care professionals we have been priviledged
to work with in their journeys of recovery. May God bless you.

Contents

Foreword

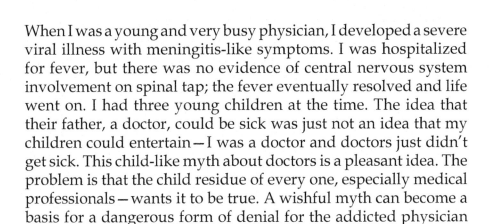

When I was a young and very busy physician, I developed a severe viral illness with meningitis-like symptoms. I was hospitalized for fever, but there was no evidence of central nervous system involvement on spinal tap; the fever eventually resolved and life went on. I had three young children at the time. The idea that their father, a doctor, could be sick was just not an idea that my children could entertain — I was a doctor and doctors just didn't get sick. This child-like myth about doctors is a pleasant idea. The problem is that the child residue of every one, especially medical professionals — wants it to be true. A wishful myth can become a basis for a dangerous form of denial for the addicted physician and his family.

It's not difficult to see how professionals can develop addictions — a biologically or psychologically vulnerable professional, exposed to sustained high performance stress, isolated by the high self expectations and those of public or loved ones, and entrusted with access to a range of dependence/ addiction inducing substances.

This book focuses uniquely on the substance dependence problems of the health professional — the healer — their diagnosis, elements of both successful and unsuccessful treatment, the generally optimistic outcome of their treatment as well as factors that militate against the overall positive treatment outcome. The goals of treatment need to go well beyond the withdrawal and avoidance of addicting substances and activities; it must help establish new and healthy reinforcements in life. The evidence is presented indicating that once a health professional enters treatment, the prognosis is often positive. Psychiatric comorbidity and especially premature discontinuation of follow-up treatment are shown to be predictors of poor outcome.

Although the data making up this book relate directly to the treatment of the addicted healer, many of the principles arising from the authors' experiences can be seen as important in any individual entrusted with the responsibility of living a decent life. In this sense, the data and conclusions can be generalized. The overall message is one of great hope—given the diagnosis and treatment program, not only a career, or a family, but a life can be saved. This book provides guideposts toward this lifesaving intervention for those who need it, their friends, and families.

Jan Fawcett, M.D. Stanley G. Harris,
Sr. Department of Psychiatry
Rush-Presbyterian–St. Luke's Medical Center

Acknowledgments

Daniel Angres, M.D., and Kathy Bettinarcli-Angres, M.S., R.N., representing Rush Behavioral Health, and G. Douglas Talbott, M.D., representing Talbott Recovery Campus, wish to acknowledge the staff of both institutions. Dr. Daniel Angres would also like to acknowledge the former Parkside Medical Services organizations. It is their efforts that are reflected in so much of this book. The authors are also indebted to their patients for whom we exist. We extend heartfelt appreciation to our families: the Angres, Talbotts, and Bettinardis.

Particular acknowledgment should be made to state medical societies/ Physician Health Committees and their leaders whose pioneering efforts have assisted so many physicians in their recovery.

Several doctors contributed to these chapters and we wish to gratefully acknowledge them: Drs. Tom Porter, Howard Kravitz, and John Oldershaw. Special thanks to Dr. Jan Fawcett, Ben Underwood, and the American Society of Addiction Medicine.

The authors Daniel H. Angres and Kathy Bettinardi-Angres would like to make a special acknowledgment to Dr. Douglas G. Talbott. He has been a loyal and cherished friend, a spiritual guide, and enlightened mentor for both of us.

Preface

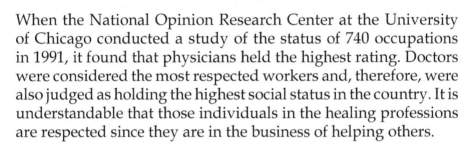

When the National Opinion Research Center at the University of Chicago conducted a study of the status of 740 occupations in 1991, it found that physicians held the highest rating. Doctors were considered the most respected workers and, therefore, were also judged as holding the highest social status in the country. It is understandable that those individuals in the healing professions are respected since they are in the business of helping others.

Even with the increase in malpractice and decrease in positive public opinion, people still admire doctors and other professional caregivers, but the health care professions are made up of human beings. Medical professionals become sick, get divorced, and become chemically dependent. Their high social status contributes to something we call the "M-Deity Syndrome": Physicians and other medical professionals are looked at as if they were gods, and, gradually, many begin to accept this role. The syndrome can cause problems with job performance, family life, and the medical marriage and can contribute to chemical dependency.

Health care professionals are often comforted by the accolades of patients and colleagues, and problems such as chemical dependency are ignored or enabled. The denial and shame increase, making it more difficult to acknowledge personal problems, leading to a conspiracy of silence. Unfortunately, the health care provider becomes sicker, sometimes suicidal, and patient care can be compromised.

Helping others is common to physicians, nurses, dentists, pharmacists, and others in the health care field. It is this caretaking role that allows the authors to universalize intervention and treatment specifications for physicians to other healers. Special considerations once employed for physicians are now working for other professionals in highly accountable positions. In this book, the focus is on the physician, but the term *healer* includes all health care professionals.

We will discuss chemical dependency as a disease and examine how we can intervene as colleagues, family members, or even patients. We will also look at how chemical dependency affects those close to the health professional. Chemical dependency is the same disease in all people, but the nature of the work of doctors and health professionals creates a specific problem that requires specific methods and resources to treat it. Physicians are no strangers to responsibility, but recovering doctors and health professionals need to be reminded that as human beings they can receive care and healing as well. They need to know they are not alone.

Kathy Bettinardi-Angres

Introduction

A HISTORICAL PERSPECTIVE

by G. Douglas Talbott, M.D.

The course of chemical dependency in the life of a health care professional can be followed by taking a historical perspective from my life story. I would like to share a few memorable moments in my own disease and recovery. I know from my clinical practice that many addicted and recovering health professionals will be able to empathize. Others will get a glimpse of the havoc this disease can wreak on one's life and yet experience the hope and recovery that can follow.

In 1949, after attending Yale University and Columbia Medical School, I entered a residency training program in internal medicine and cardiology. I chose the University of California in San Francisco for my training and ended my 4 years there as Chief Resident in internal medicine. In my third year of medical school, I married my wife Polly and we began our family; within 15 years, we had six children. The basic elements of my disease, however, were present during my childhood, and drinking as an adult was not only socially acceptable, but a major part of the culture. As an adult, I began to suffer from the never-addressed problems of an adult child of an alcoholic.

While I was in medical school, I began to experience panic attacks. I regarded the advent and increased severity of these episodes with terror and shame. I talked with no one about the fearful hours and days experiencing palpitations, sweating, tachycardia, anxiety, and impending doom. Large doses of alcohol, when consumed quickly, were very effective in alleviating these attacks. Where I had previously avoided alcohol because of the pain associated with my mother's alcoholism, I now began to abuse alcohol.

My career was beginning to take off and blossom. At the same time, I was hiding this awful secret and progressing in the stages of alcoholism. I founded, with the help of the James Cox family and others, the Cox Coronary Heart Institute in Dayton, Ohio, where I was born. I was widely respected, my income was above average, and I had a loving family. Yet, my life was disintegrating. My wife and I were drifting apart physically and emotionally due to my drinking. My children were confused and lost and their behavior reflected my excessive drinking. For the first time my staff and peers were questioning my behavior and judgment. The only peace I seemed to experience came when drinking. My disease progressed and I started using demerol and sedatives to supplement and complement the drinking.

When my stomach became so inflamed I could not drink, I would inject medications for relief. Alcohol was my drug of choice, however. The disease had a drastic impact on my family. Love and trust were replaced with doubt and mistrust. The outer circles of my life had already been stripped away. My community involvement, the church, relationships with colleagues, and leisure time had gradually disappeared. I had broken contact with distant family. My life became either working or using. I had peeled away everybody except Polly and my children, and toward the end, I even distanced myself from them. It is important to note that I was not drinking for fun and never enjoyed it in any stage of my disease. I drank only to stop the incredible pain. I became more isolated, and anger, mistrust, and lack of self-respect were my constant companions.

My life spiraled downward, and I was eventually fired from the Cox Institute. I was admitted to a number of psychiatric hospitals for various treatments, and yet I continued to drink. My wife never left me, but my behavior caused her to feel deep resentment, fear, and anger. This only heightened my despair and self-loathing. Then, after all other treatment attempts had failed, I was committed to Dayton State Mental Hospital. The hospital was grossly understaffed that rainy night, and the inmates of my cell, who included the criminally insane, verbally and physically tortured me. I was in withdrawal from the drugs and alcohol and too debilitated to defend myself. I will never forget lying there bleeding, in severe pain, and even suffering through the humiliation of being urinated on. I kept thinking, God, where are you? Lying on the floor that night, I clearly remember making a vow to myself that if I ever got out of this place alive, I would dedicate my life to helping doctors and other health care professionals in this situation. I vowed I would find a way to help suffering doctors like myself and dreamed of one day creating a place where healers could be healed.

After a few months of abstinence, I left the hospital. The single biggest factor in my survival was the love and support of Polly and my children. There was also a Catholic priest, Father Richard DeCavitt, who rekindled my faith in God and was responsible for helping me join Alcoholics Anonymous (AA). These were the crucial elements in the beginning of my recovery.

Father DeCavitt also guided me in my decision to leave the field of cardiology and internal medicine, and learn about the disease of alcoholism. Twenty-five years ago, the study and management of addiction did not even warrant a position in medicine. However, I studied and learned at the Addiction School in Toronto, Yale University, and Rutgers School of Alcoholism. At that time, in the summer of 1971, the director of the Maryland Program was Dr. Maxwell Weisman. He was my teacher, role model and friend over the next 3 years as I worked for him as Director of the Baltimore Public Inebriate Program. Initially, as part of my education before actually starting the job as director, I lived on the streets with other alcoholics. I did this for 9 weeks, sleeping in abandoned warehouses and panhandling with skid-row alcoholics. This experience deeply moved me and greatly influenced my future work with addicts and alcoholics. I learned the skid-row culture. For the first time in my life I was relating to people without the trappings of material goods or my titles. I only had myself to give to them and they to me. Living with the skid-row alcoholics, I gained their trust, and they taught me the cornerstones of recovery: honesty, love, and sharing.

I spent 3 years in Baltimore, and during the last 2 years, I began to assist the Maryland State Medical Society in planning a program for impaired physicians. This was the very beginning of the impaired physicians movement. The Georgia program was initiated after our National Institutes of Health (NIH) grant ran out in Baltimore. Dr. Oscar Vinson, the DeKalb Health Director in Atlanta, persuaded me to take a job there. When I determined that the Medical Association of Georgia had a positive and caring attitude toward impaired physicians, I started the Georgia Impaired Physicians Program at the Georgia Clinic, which was later called the DeKalb Addiction Clinic.

The Georgia Program initially treated patients with an inpatient hospitalization followed by an outpatient phase. It was apparent, however, that the patients needed extended treatment. I moved the center to a metropolitan hospital and included family counseling and an aftercare group with a focus on physicians called a Caduceus Club.'[2] The Caduceus Clubs have grown and expanded to more than 90 in number across North America. I

---

2 ' The Caduceus meetings were established 23 years ago with an objective of allowing physicians and ultimately other health professionals to gather and share their experiences of recovery from the diseases of chemical dependence and other addictions. Initially, these meetings were confined to the Atlanta area and limited to graduates of the Talbott Recovery Campus who were all physicians. However, in the past three decades, there have evolved 90 Caduceus Clubs throughout the United States and Canada. Constituency

expanded the residential facilities by renting apartments throughout the Atlanta area. I also started an experimental training program called "Mirror-Image Therapy." Recovering physicians and other health care professionals participated as counselor trainees in alcoholism and addiction. They would sit across the table and ask their patients, "Can't you see what you're doing to your family?" and they would see a mirror image of themselves. This was an invaluable method for them to gain insight into their own lives. Family therapy was recognized as an invaluable part of recovery, and a multiphased extensive family therapy program was developed. With Ben Lenderwood I developed the doctor's program at the Talbott Recovery Campus.

I soon was crisscrossing the United States to meet with graduates who were starting programs of their own. One of these graduates is Dr. Daniel Angres, who began a treatment program in Illinois in 1984. Every year since has seen the growth of the Georgia and Illinois programs. There is still a critical need for education, identification, intervention, and treatment of health care professionals in this country. The authors of this book feel it is time to document our collective experiences in order to better serve a highly misunderstood and dangerous disease. Our goal is to share our experiences, research, and stories to provide health professionals, their families, and their associates with a map of recovery.

---

now includes, in many clubs, all health professionals. The format varies from discussion meetings to 12-step programs.

The Caduceus meetings cannot be substituted for or confused with Alcoholics Anonymous or other 12-step programs. Rather, the Caduceus meetings are a bridge for many recovering health professionals into AA, NA, or CA, or other 12-step programs. In some rural areas, the Caduceus Clubs now include recovering people outside of the health care professionals.

THE FUTURE

The treatment and recovery of alcoholic and addicted health care professionals is of great interest to society today.

With the influx of new mood-altering chemicals, the increasing abuse of alcohol and drugs by young people, and the heightened fear and intolerance of others in our society, this disease needs to be in the forefront of medicine. Physicians, nurses, dentists, pharmacists, and others in highly accountable professions are already under the microscope. When they are diagnosed with the disease of chemical dependency, society turns a critical eye and hope for the future dims. The personal lives of the authors have been enhanced in the recovery, so we feel optimistic. But, the reality is that society does not have the same experience. Education and compassion appear to be the keys for reaching an understanding and alleviating fear of any disease or mental illness. We hope this book will provide readers with increased knowledge and leave them with a sense of hope and optimism about the future. Health professionals are natural role models, and their experience with chemical dependency, one hopes, can pave the way for others' success in recovery. Health professionals can be models as well as modelers. Recovering physicians with good sobriety touch the lives of many people. This ripple effect has a vast and powerful influence in the field of addiction medicine. The American Society of Addiction Medicine (ASAM), the addiction arm of the American Medical Association (AMA), has come to play a powerful role for the impaired physician.

1

The Disease of Chemical Dependency

Despite scientific evidence, some health care professionals have difficulty accepting the precept that addiction is a primary disease entity. However, in the last two decades, our knowledge regarding chemical dependency as a complex disease has allowed us to accept the primary disease precept for chemical dependency.

Historically, chemical dependency was often seen as a sign of underlying psychopathology rather than as a primary disease entity. Efforts were made to "correct" the underlying psychopathology with the hope that the secondary chemical dependency would disappear. These efforts had particularly poor outcomes. Today, we recognize chemical dependency not only as a disease state, but as a primary disease with established etiologic agents or causes and a recognizable set of signs and symptoms that permit accurate diagnosis and a predictable, progressive course. We also recognize that chemical dependency is a complex disease state that includes biogenetic and psychosocial phenomena. When the "stress diathesis" concept of addiction as a disease is applied, chemical dependency typically involves biogenetic risk factors that make an individual particularly vulnerable to chemicals (diathesis). Consequently, environmental factors, such as early developmental issues, concomitant psychiatric illness, peer pressure, work, and family discord (stress), may trigger the primary symptom of chemical dependency—the compulsive use of mood altering, addicting chemicals (MACs) despite adverse consequences.

After concentrated study, the American Society of Addiction Medicine and the National Council of Alcoholism and Drug Dependency have arrived at a definition of alcoholism. This definition applies to other drug addictions as well.

> Alcoholism is a primary, chronic disease with genetic, psychosocial, and environmental factors influencing its development and manifestation. The disease is also progressive and fatal. It is characterized by continuous or periodic impaired control over drinking, preoccupation with the drug alcohol, use of alcohol despite adverse consequences, and distortions in thinking, most notably denial. (Morse & Flavin, 1992, pp. 1012-1014)

Dependency does not automatically occur with all individuals who use chemicals. In fact, the majority of individuals who use MACs appear to be able to take or leave the substances rather than become compulsively involved with their use. Our observations strongly suggest that chemical dependency is far more than a physiologic addiction. In fact, it is the distinctive heightened experience that occurs in the chemically dependent person that drives the addiction. This experience is produced by a complex process combining unique alterations in neurochemistry with the specific properties of the chemical to which one is most sensitive, and it is far more profound than what the substance itself should inherently produce. The heightened experience may not only be euphoric, but as the disease progresses it becomes freedom from pain in the emotional, physical, and situational sense.

The concept of a lock and key helps to illustrate this unique phenomenon. The lock (also referred to as "broken filter") is the sum of neurochemical alterations from genetic causes as well as a series of environmental factors—early developmental and external stressors, for example—that yield a predisposition to the effects of MACs. The key is the substance (for both neurochemical and psychological reasons) that unlocks this dramatic experience. It is this experience that helps drive the compulsive use of the substance despite adverse consequences. Although this broken filter is perhaps more sensitive to a specific class of drug in any given individual, it is vulnerable to all MACs. Here the concept of cross-addition is critical. Even a drug that does not produce this experience but is mood-altering and addicting can become a new drug of choice or produce a series of neurochemical alterations that eventually will lead back to the original drug of choice and the resultant loss of control. For example, someone whose drug of choice is cocaine may rationalize that they never got out of control with alcohol. During recovery from cocaine addiction, they attempt to use alcohol socially and find that in a short period of time they are back on cocaine.

THE DISEASE SPECTRUM

Alcoholism was described as a disease as early as the 1950s by the American Medical Association. Unfortunately, the psychiatric literature too often represented dependence on other mood-altering chemicals such as opiates, amphetamines, and minor tranquilizers as symptoms of an underlying psychopathology. Today, we recognize that chemical dependency is truly a continuum that involves dependence on all mood-altering chemicals. Whether a drug is legal or illegal, socially acceptable or unacceptable, has nothing to do with central nervous system functioning and the response to the chemicals in the disease state. All mood-altering, addicting substances are part of a continuum. Although different, with some classes of drugs affecting specific neurotransmitters more than others, all MACs will produce the compulsive loss of control in vulnerable individuals.

In recent years, there has been discussion about other addictive behaviors such as compulsive gambling, overeating, or even sexual acting out as constituting part of the disease spectrum beyond chemical dependency. These are commonly described as process addictions. Today, we are thinking in terms of what we call addictive spectrum illness. This spectrum represents a series of variations on a common theme. Whether it is a chemical or a behavior that is consistently abused, the end result can be the same — loss of control with lethal or destructive consequences.

Chemical abuse is defined as a maladaptive pattern of drug use, including alcohol, leading to significant impairment or distress manifested by one or more of the following elements:

- Failure to fulfill major roles at home or work.
- Recurrent drug or alcohol use in situations in which it is physically hazardous (i.e., driving motorized vehicles, flying aircraft, etc.).
- Recurrent drug or alcohol-related legal problems (i.e., DUIs/DWIs, disorderly conduct, etc.).
- Drug or alcohol use while rendering patient care.
- Continued drug or alcohol use despite persistent social or interpersonal problems caused or exacerbated by the effects of the drugs or alcohol.

DEFINITION OF CHEMICAL DEPENDENCY

Too often, chemical abuse has been confused with chemical dependency. Abuse has been described as the use of MACs for a specific period of time with eventual physical consequences (but without compulsion). Chemical dependency is very different from abuse. Chemical dependency, while including abuse and the recognition of loss of control, has other specific characteristics.

Tolerance and withdrawal are two important conditions associated with chemical dependency. Tolerance is essentially the need for more of the substance in order to get the same desired effect. Withdrawal is a clear-cut physiologic response that occurs with the abrupt cessation of use of a MAC by someone who has become physiologically dependent. Although tolerance and withdrawal are often present in chemically dependent people, addiction to alcohol and MACs may have no specific relationship to tolerance and withdrawal. This, however, can also be seen in nonaddicted people such as patients on an oncology unit. Addiction certainly occurs in the absence of observable tolerance with withdrawal (Miller, Dackis, & Gold, 1987). A much more complete definition of chemical dependency must highlight the compulsive components of the disease, recognizing that continued substance use, despite persistent, recurrent, and adverse consequences in an individual's social, financial, psychological, or physical life, is one of the major factors in chemical dependency.

NEUROTRANSMITTER FUNCTIONS

Understanding chemical dependency requires an understanding of some of the primary risk factors, including neurochemical factors. Neurotransmitters are brain messengers that provide communication between one brain cell and another across a space called the synaptic cleft. Major groups of neurotransmitters include dopamine, norepinephrine, serotonin, gamma-amino-butyric acid (GAM), acetylcholine, endorphins, and enkephalins. These neurotransmitters can account for most of the symptoms seen with the drugs most commonly abused in the United States (Giannini & Miller, 1989). Different MACs affect different neurotransmitters. For example, it is thought that GABA is most sensitive to sedative hypnotics, including alcohol, barbiturates, and minor tranquilizers. Acetylcholine is particularly sensitive to phencyclidine. Norepinephrine is most affected by amphetamines and other stimulants such as cocaine, but it is also in a feedback loop with opiates. Dopamine is the primary neurotransmitter affected by cocaine, but amphetamines and phencyclidine affect dopamine as well. Opiates inhibit GABA that in turn leads to dopamine release (Leshner, 1996). Serotonin, in part, can be influenced by psychedelic agents, cocaine, and perhaps even alcohol. Endorphins and enkephalins are known to be affected by opiates but are also thought to be affected by many MACs, including alcohol.

HOW NEUROTRANSMITTERS AFFECT US

We know today that most MACs will produce an initial response that reflects the heightened activity of the affected neurotransmitter. This happens when the substances block the reuptake of specific neurotransmitters or actually produce greater release. In any case, the greater the amount of neurotransmitters affected, the greater the response produced. However, if a MAC is used repeatedly, either intermittently as in a binge pattern or chronically as in a continuous use pattern, neurotransmitter release is eventually slowed, and finally, the neurotransmitters affected are depleted. This produces cravings and dysphoria.

Neurotransmitters have considerable effects on our mood. We suspect that some conditions, such as schizophrenia, represent an excess of certain neurotransmitters such as dopamine. Depletion of some neurotransmitters, such as norepinephrine or serotonin, plays a critical role in major depressive illness and other psychiatric disorders. MACs, in affecting these neurotransmitters by transiently increasing them to the point of eventual depletion, can clearly give rise to severe psychiatric symptoms. Often these symptoms mimic psychiatric illness.

These neurochemical changes, along with the destruction of defense mechanisms (the consequence of isolation, etc.), produce a series of psychiatric phenomena, such as confusional states, depression, and anxiety, that are often diagnosed as primary psychiatric conditions. However, many psychiatric symptoms produced by chemical dependency are secondary phenomena or symptoms of the chemical dependency rather than of psychiatric illness.

Different neurotransmitters are clearly targeted by different MACs. However, there is certainly a link among all neurotransmitter systems. An individual's drug of choice may be in part influenced by how the different neurotransmitters are programed in terms of the particular person's vulnerability to specific MACs.

CHRONIC ABUSE OF ALCOHOL AND DRUGS

Although we have a good understanding of how neurotransmitters function and which MACs will affect which neurotransmitters, we have less understanding of the common denominators that neurochemically predispose an individual to chemical dependency. Obviously, we can see by neurotransmitter function that the effect of limited use or abuse is much different from that of chronic use. But why do some people become involved with the continued abuse of substances despite the adverse consequences (such as those seen as a result of the disease of chemical dependency) while most people who use chemicals do not lose control?

This question has resulted in much study regarding how genetics, and perhaps other factors (e.g., early development), can influence neurochemistry prior to the use of MACs (Noble, 1991; Tarter, Hegedus, Goldstein, Shelly, & Alterman, 1984).

There has been a great deal of interest in research involving internal opiates, such as endorphins and enkephalins, and their receptors. We know that stress can deplete our internal opiates

(Blum et al., 1990). It is even conceivable that part of what is genetically influenced is a relative reduction in internal opiates or receptor responsivity (Faraj et al., 1987). Blum and Payne (1991) described a somatopsychic theory that establishes a link among genes, brain chemistry, and behavior. Certain genes can ultimately regulate the neurotransmitters responsible for a feeling of well-being. If these genes are defective, different conditions, including cravings, compulsion, and drug-seeking behavior, can occur. It can be stated that the user and abuser drink for pleasure, the addict and alcoholic drug and drink to alleviate pain, and at times, withdrawal symptoms.

Dopamine appears to play a major role within the brain's reward mechanisms critical to compulsive usage patterns, much like that of electrical brain stimulation reward. The self-administration of drugs activates the same brain reward mechanisms including the mesolimbic DA system that runs through the medial forebrain bundle (Gardner, 1992). Recently, the National Institute of Drug Abuse acknowledged drug addiction as a "brain disease," noting positron emission tomography (PET) findings, including persistent decrease in metabolic function of the mesolimbic DA system after chemical use (Leshner, 1996).

The reward phenomena in the brain interact in complex patterns resembling a cascade. For example, serotonin stimulates enkephalin and inhibits GABA, releasing dopamine, which activates dopaminergic receptors; this produces feelings of well-being (Blum & Payne, 1991). Disturbances in this cascade could create problems with those feelings of well-being and trigger cravings and compulsion (Blum & Trachtenberg, 1987).

A genetically induced reduction or relative loss of responsiveness of our internal opiates, precipitated by abuse, would make one more sensitive to euphoria-producing substances (e.g., drugs and alcohol) . Since alcohol, opiates, and mood-altering substances in general can influence these opiate receptors, a relative deficiency in these neurochemicals could mean heightened response to externally administered euphoria-producing chemicals. However, since MACS eventually deplete our own neurotransmitters, a vicious cycle would be produced. A dramatic response to use of an external MAC would occur since it is supplementing what we suspect is an initially deficient state before the chemical use. It is characterized as "running two quarts low" on internally produced "feel-good" chemistry (i.e., endorphins, dopamine, and other neurotransmitters).

When an MAC from the outside interacts with the receptors of these neurotransmitters, a transient but powerful sense of well-being, or at least freedom from pain, unique to the chemically dependent person, is felt. This may provide an understanding of the magical experience that is described by chemically dependent people when they "connect" with their drug of choice. In fact, recognizing that the power of this experience is what drives the chemically dependent person to lose control is essential to understanding chemical dependency. It is the unique neurochemistry and psychology of the addict combined with the properties inherent in the chemical itself that produce the addict's enhanced experience with his or her drug of choice.

This leads to unusual reactions to certain chemicals among chemically dependent people. For example, it is not uncommon to see someone with an opiate dependence become energized by opiates, although typically these drugs produce sedation. This happens in many chemically dependent people whose drug of choice is alcohol or other seda- tive hypnotics. Conversely, those chemically dependent people whose drugs of choice are stimulants often describe "mellowing" when using their drug of choice.

These paradoxical responses are typical in chemically dependent people. This magical experience unique to the chemically dependent person is often described not only as a powerful sense of well-being, but also as a feeling of being "normalized," a freedom from discomfort, anhedonia, or dysphoria, rather than of becoming inordinately high from the substances (Angres & Benson, 1985). After this typically short-lived experience, reduction of the intensity of the experience leads to increased use often to the point of toxicity. The more one uses, the more one's internal chemistry depletes; the more one depletes, the more one craves, and so on. This vicious cycle continues to deplete internal opiates and/ or dopamine stores. These unique responses, or this magical experience, may be due to internal opioid metabolism or, perhaps, to other neurotransmitter metabolisms such as the dopaminergic system or a combination of multiple systems (Wise, 1987).

GENETICS

It has been shown that genetics clearly contribute to the vulnerability of certain individuals to MACs. A considerable amount of research has been done with alcohol, but what is true for alcoholism also holds true for other substances in this spectrum (Miller & Chappel, 1991). Family illness studies, twin studies, and adoption studies have been three major areas of genetic study for alcoholism.

Family illness studies have shown that the offspring of chemically dependent parents are more vulnerable to alcoholism (Schuckit, 1981). Twin studies have demonstrated that identical twins, who share the same gene pool, as opposed to fraternal twins, who share only 50%, have a higher concordance rate for alcoholism (Schuckit, 1985). That is to say, when alcoholism is present in the family, identical twins will be more vulnerable than fraternal twins.

The argument of nature versus nurture has been addressed by adoption studies. It was shown that adopted children whose biological parents were alcoholics had a four-times higher risk for alcoholism than a control group (Goodwin, Schulsinger, Moller, Hermansen, Winoker, & Guze, 1974).

In these studies, it was suggested that a person's biologic or genetic influences were stronger determinants of whether they would become chemically dependent than were events in their early development. As with many common illnesses and diseases, chemical dependency appears to rely on the interaction between biological—genetic factors, use of addictive chemicals, and environmental exposure (Dinwiddie & Cloninger, 1991). Further evidence of this has been shown by studies suggesting that very specific manifestations of alcohol abuse seem to be genetically linked as well. For example, there appears to be a genetic predisposition to a syndrome such as Wernicke's encephalopathy caused by an abnormality in the enzyme system regarding thiamine metabolism (Reuler, Girard, & Cooney, 1985).

More recently, some dramatic studies have suggested that there is a specific observable genetic abnormality. Allelic association of a dopamine D2 receptor gene has been described in blood samples obtained from alcoholics and their relatives, but was not present in nonalcoholic samples (Blum et al., 1990). The identification of a possible gene for alcoholism is an exciting development since it might lead to the possibility of early identification. Other research has suggested that low platelet monoamine oxidase activity among alcoholics may provide other biochemical markers for alcoholism (Faraj et al., 1987). Not only is genetic research in chemical dependency now providing documentation of the importance of inherited factors in this disease, but in the future it also may provide a critically important means of prevention and early identification of this disease.

ADDICTIVE PERSONALITY

Growing evidence suggests that chemical dependency is more than simply the biologically mediated heightened response to MACs in the susceptible host. A good deal of discussion has occurred regarding premorbid personality types that are influenced by both genetic and early developmental elements (see Chapter 10).

Earlier trait studies suggested that depression and sociopathy were the two most common character traits found in the chemically dependent person (Weismann & Myers, 1980; Woodruff, Guze, Clayton, & Carr, 1973). More recent research has documented that these retrospective studies simply confirmed that while antisocial behavior and depression are often the consequences of chemical dependence, they are not inherent traits in chemically dependent people. The 12 steps and 12 traditions in the "Big Book" or *Alcoholics Anonymous* (1976) make many references to an addictive style of functioning. Traditional psychiatry has discussed narcissistic personality defects in chemically dependent people. It also was suggested by the psychoanalytic communities that chemical dependency occurs in those individuals who, because of difficulties in early development, have problems with ego strength. With the loss of ego strength, they said, the addiction-prone individual seeks nurturing from the outside because of difficulty in producing the experiences internally. Others suggest that individuals with different drugs of choice have different personality subtypes. For example, stimulus hunger seen in cocaine-dependent individuals suggests that these subtypes, along with their drugs of choice, were mediated by different neurotransmitter systems (in this case, dopamine).

Other studies have suggested that the offspring of chemically dependent parents, as compared with control groups, have a higher rate of attention-deficit disorder, problems with mood regulation, and even changes in brain-wave functions (Tarter et al., 1984). It has been our observation that there are indeed a variety of addictive personalities, and that these personalities are not an indication of some underlying psychopathology, but are part of the process of the disease of chemical dependency. These personalities are variable and tend toward problems with anxiety, impulsiveness, and poor self-esteem. This anxiety can best be described as a heightened sensitivity to the addict's environment. Through chemical use, the addict attempts to modify and dampen that sensitivity. Impulsiveness, with difficulty in delaying gratification, is the hallmark of a chemically dependent personality profile. Problems with self-esteem certainly can plague anyone, but it appears that chemically dependent people have greater problems in this area. The need for a healthy self-concept, one that is not defensively grandiose or reactively low, is critical for recovery.

RISK FACTORS

We now begin to develop a model for the disease of chemical dependency. As mentioned earlier in this chapter, the idea of stress diathesis plays an important role in creating this model; that is, there is a biogenetic susceptibility in the host that combines with both internal and external environmental factors. This can be represented in an $X + Y = Z$ formula. X is the biogenetic risk factor — the genetically induced, neurochemically vulnerable state that results in an enhanced experience with substances.

The Y factor involves both internal and external environmental stressors. These include developmental issues, such as responses to neglect in early childhood, leading to narcissism and other character deficits. The Y factor certainly also includes the tendency toward depression or anxiety. Individuals with true concomitant psychiatric illness, as we see in dual diagnoses, would be at a greater risk if this were also part of the Y factor. Additionally, exposure to and abuse of MACs in the environment is a major risk. Peer influence plays a significant role in this factor, as does society's general adherence to a "chemical culture," indicated by the acceptance of MAC use as a critical part of the ability to celebrate life. Other social and environmental factors can include job stress, marital or other relationship discord, chronic pain syndrome, or specific situational stress.

In our equation, Z is the disease of chemical dependency. In the biogenetically susceptible individual (X), exposure and abuse of the chemicals themselves, as well as both psychological and social stresses (1') , will sooner or later lead to the use of MACs despite adverse consequences — in other words, loss of control. Variations within this simple formula, regarding primary risk factors and mediating conditions leading to the final expression of the illness of alcoholism, have been well studied (Donovan, 1986).

Finally, a case can also be made for $Y - X = Z$ equation. Here there is no perceivable presence of biogenetic predisposition, but there is a predominance of Y factors unduly influencing a given individual to use MACs. Consequently, the heightened experience, or magical connection, would not be the primary experience. For example, someone who has chronic pain and is treated by the long-term use of MACs such as opiates will then become physically and psychologically dependent on them. At some point, that individual will begin to depend on the chemical to obtain not only pain management but also the experience produced by the substance. We understand that drugs are powerful reinforcers with or without physical dependence (Meisch, 1991). In a case like this, the treatment would be unlikely to differ from the $X + Y = Z$ formally, since the experience has become ingrained. The prognosis may be better since the inherent vulnerability and even premorbid addictive personality style would not be a factor; however, too often we see chemical dependency occurring in individuals who have both the X factor and the chronic pain syndrome, contributing to the X factor. In this case, subtyping seems to play an important role in chemically dependent individuals in terms of where they might be in this spectrum with a predominance of X factors at one extreme and the influence of Y factors at the other.

SUBTYPING THE X FACTOR

Cloninger (1987), in his discussion of neurogenetic adaptive mechanisms of alcoholism, describes subtypes 1 and 2. Subtype 1 involves individuals described as late-onset alcoholics. They often have a history of controllable alcohol use, but later in life begin to exhibit loss of control, typically in a binge-type pattern. This may represent a predominance of Y factors superimposed on lesser X factors. In these instances, a threshold is reached and the disease becomes apparent.

Subtype 2 involves early onset and continuous use of MACs, with enhanced tolerance for the substances, leading to rapid escalation of the disease with a broad range of consequences. This type may represent the other side of the spectrum where X factors play a predominant role. Here, the first exposure to the chemical often produces the connection immediately and initiates a rapid progression of the disease. It is thought that male offspring of type 2 alcoholic fathers have a 9-times increased incidence of alcoholism, suggesting a strong genetic basis or predominance for this subtype.

ISOLATION AND NEED FOR BONDING

The ability for intimacy with or without chemicals during the active course of the disease is greatly impaired. Severe isolation produces the use of maladaptive and regressed defense mechanisms and relationships suffer as a consequence. Even from a neurochemical standpoint, primate research has shown that isolation directly affects the number and sensitivity of opiate receptors (Coe, Glass, Weiner, & Levine, 1983) as well as other neurotransmitter systems. Whether employing a psychological, social, or biogenetic model, or a combination of all of these factors, one cannot ignore the tragic destruction that occurs in chemically dependent people in terms of their internal resources and their ability to meaningfully bond with others.

Treatment for this disease not only requires the commitment to abstinence and the strategies necessary to maintain abstinence from MACs, but also must include strategies for true recovery; that is, the ability to replace MACs with health-enhancing entities. Primary to all of this is the need for bonding with other human beings.

The most powerful experience of all should be the experience of the healthy, human encounter, not chemical experience. Bonding with others and the need for self-exploration and understanding are essential to recovery. The ability to better understandoneself and the triggers that surround one is essential. We have found no better vehicle for this ability to know oneself and bond with others than the group process, leading ultimately to immersion in a 12-step program (e.g., Alcoholics Anonymous) .

Additionally, AA's program brings in the essential element of a spiritual focus. In the downward spiral of addiction, the addict becomes absorbed with self to the exclusion of all else, including a sense of a higher power. The substances replace, and then become, the higher power.

A HOLISTIC APPROACH

Recovery involves a holistic approach to life. In addition to the ability to know oneself, bond with others, and gain recognition of a higher power, other nonchemical coping skills must be developed. Development of a healthy diet with minimal caffeine and elimination of nicotine should be included here. Nicotine addiction is a major health hazard, and its treatment is often addressed concurrently with chemical dependency treatment. However, because nicotine initially produces minimal mood-altering effects, but can result in severe withdrawal symptoms, it only partially fits the disease model discussed here. Use of over-the-counter (OTC) drugs needs to be carefully evaluated for MAC content. Exercise is a critical factor not only in maintaining good cardiovascular fitness and general health, but also in mobilizing the endorphin and enkephalin systems, which are suspected to be deficient in chemically dependent people even prior to the use of chemicals. And finally, meditation, in any form, gives one the ability to get in touch with a quieter place with fewer distractions, and therefore to become closer to a source within that can keep one centered and serene.

Referring to the earlier mentioned model of a depleted dopamine, endorphin, and enkephalin system as being one of the essential elements that may contribute to the X factor, one might suspect that chemically dependent individuals will have trouble mobilizing their feel-good capacities, even after becoming abstinent from chemicals. However, a feedback loop in that neurochemistry (endorphins, enkephalins, dopamine, or other neurotransmitters) affects our feeling states and behavior, and our behavior and feeling states affect our neurochemistry. Many studies, including primate studies, suggest that the brain has "structural plasticity" and is influenced by pathologic states as well as by psychosocial factors and even psychotherapy (Gabbard, 1992).

There is no permanent way to readjust our neurochemistry or addictive personality tendencies. Elimination of all stressors will not do it. A daily program of abstinence and the use of non-chemical coping skills are the only means to recovery. As recovery progresses, one can grow spiritually, emotionally, and even neurochemically in ways that were unavailable before the use of the chemicals. Through adherence to a strong program, a gift can come with recovery, namely, that through the pain of this disease one can develop a way of life and true sobriety that is increasingly fulfilling and satisfying.

SUMMARY

The disease of chemical dependency is a complex process involving biogenetic and psychosocial risk factors. Current scientific evidence supports the theory that chemical dependency tends to occur in individuals who are biogenetically predisposed to the specific effects of MACs. Once exposed to and abusing these chemicals, for both psychological and social reasons, the individual experiences them in a way that eventually leads to their compulsive use. In turn, the susceptible host continues to use the chemicals despite the adverse consequences that characterize chemical dependency.

We are learning more about the complex process of genetically induced neurochemical changes, with particular interest in the dopamine, endorphin, and enkephalin systems. Growing evidence supports the idea that there is an addictive personality style that may include a tendency toward anxiety, impulsiveness, and problems with self-esteem. There are also indications that an individual predisposed to this disease might experience a lack of dopamine, internal opiates, or feel-good chemical capacity. As noted earlier, this has been described as running two quarts low on internally produced feel-good chemistry. The gift of sobriety allows individuals to remain abstinent through the use of various nonchemical coping skills, and most importantly, to bond with others in a group and in a 12-step program. This not only provides spiritual, emotional, and psychological wellbeing, but also provides the ability to mobilize these feel-good chemicals beyond their original resting state. Abstinence is avoidance of MACs and by itself is not recovery. Sobriety starts with abstinence but also includes the elements mentioned above in the gifts of sobriety.

The recovery precept clearly indicates that complete, lifelong abstinence from all MACs is the first crucial step for all those afflicted with this disease. Equally critical is the replacement of chemicals with healthy relationships and nonchemical coping skills, which are essential to transform abstinence into sobriety.

2

Chemical Dependency Treatment

THE RUSH BEHAVIORAL HEALTH AND TALBOTT RECOVERY CAMPUS PROGRAMS

The need for specialized treatment for chemically dependent health care professionals has been a major subject of discussion for several years. These professionals by definition work in highly accountable positions in the health care field; they include physicians, nurses, dentists, pharmacists, therapists, and others who are licensed in some capacity to provide patient care. The need for early intervention, individualized and often intensive treatment, and extended aftercare monitoring is often indicated when dealing with providers whose well-being directly affects the general safety and well-being of the community. This process has allowed the majority of chemically dependent health care professionals to attain sobriety and return to the workforce as healthy, competent practitioners.

[2]Whether the health care professional can be treated in the nonspecialized treatment program, either on an inpatient or outpatient basis, needs to be addressed. There is no doubt that there are health care professionals who may simply be able to get into a 12-step recovery program and bypass the formalized treatment process completely. There are others who may need long-term recovery programs as a result of the nonspecialized treatment (e.g., 3-5-week inpatient stays with a 3-month follow-up without any specialized peer-group support). In the authors' experience, however, the majority of health care professionals need longer treatment that includes specialized phases, peer-group support, and a structured long-term monitoring system. This partially holds true for patients with comorbidity, previous failures with short term treatments, and/or those who experience consequences of their disease apparent in the work place. In addition, the use of specialized-phase treatment and intensive long-term monitoring in a peer setting act as additional safeguards. Not only are health care professionals and their families being assisted, but measures are taken to maintain accountability, which helps to secure the health and wellbeing of future patients of the chemically dependent health care professional as well.

The authors' experience indicates that most chemically dependent health care professionals need a strong peer-group setting both in the initial treatment process and in long-term aftercare. The addicted professional needs not only a peer-group setting of other patients with the same disease process, but also one comprising fellow health care professionals. This helps to confront more effectively and empathetically the grandiosity,

---

2   Dr. Howard Kravitz, a contributing author to this chapter, is an Associate Professor, Departments of Psychiatry and Preventive Medicine, Rush Medical College, Chicago, Illinois; and Adjunct Associate Professor, Division of Epidemiology and Biostatistics, School of Public Health, University of Illinois at Chicago

defensiveness, and denial that are typically seen in the health care professional than would be possible in a general setting.

Denial is a major defense mechanism of victims of the disease of chemical dependency, particularly those in the health care profession. The denial of symptoms of chemical dependency not only allows for continued use of the chemicals, but also keeps addicted professionals from viewing their impairment with the proper sense of professional accountability. Health care professionals are particularly fearful of the consequences of chemical dependency on their professional lives, and will understandably defend against the idea that anything is interfering with their capabilities. The possibility that patient care could suffer or that one's ability to practice one's profession may be impaired often reinforces denial and minimization of the problem. Denial as a defense mechanism is typically most effectively confronted by other health care professionals who are in a similar circumstance.

In addition to the peergroup setting, longer phase treatment is often indicated for the health care professional, with extended aftercare. These advocacy programs are committed to health professionals' return to work.

A FOUR-PHASE TREATMENT PROCESS

The following phases, in general, reflect the treatment approach initially developed by the Talbott program, with some modifications by the Rush program (Table 2-1). The Talbott model comes from an original 4-month model that included: (1) 1 month of residential rehabilitation; (2) residing in an independent living setting; (3) attending the day hospital setting in the second month; and (4) 2 months of mirror-image placement therapy (while remaining in the apartment setting). This basic model has clearly influenced what is now a more flexible model at both the Talbott and Rush programs.

There are some different approaches between the Talbott and Rush programs:

Phase I. Both Rush and Talbott have modified the Phase I evaluation and stabilization phase to be more flexible rather than adhering to a strict 28-day model, and have even bypassed it when not clinically indicated. Average hospital stay is now 4 to 7 days, if indicated.

Table 2-1.

Phases of Treatment

Phase I	Phase II	Phase III	Phase IV
(Variable duration)	(9-6 weeks)	(9-8 weeks)	(20 months)
Diagnostic evaluation Day or evening hospital	Day or evening hospital	Mirror image/ placement phase	Extended aftercare
Determine need for treatment	Peer group setting	"Senior patient" role	Weekly monitoring and support groups
Determine initial level of care	Emphasis on primary care goals (e.g., working through denial, exploring triggers)	Examine own needs vs. needs of others	Significant-other weekly support groups
Detoxification, stabilization, and continued inpatient/ residential treatment when indicated		Can transition back to work	12-step meetings with sponsorship
	Availability of concomitant independent living program		Random urine monitoring
			Bimonthly meetings with primary physician
			Medical society interface

Phase II. In the Rush program, Phase II has the additional component of an intensive evening outpatient setting, in part because of its sizable regional patient population.

Phase III. The mirror-image placement phase involves working in some area of chemical dependency within 17 private and public sites in the greater Atlanta metropolitan area while remaining in the recovery residence in the Talbott program. In Illinois, Phase III is completed primarily at the Rush facility itself and at other Rush Behavioral Health sites.

Phase W. This phase is essentially the same at both settings and, in the cases of out-of-state patients, similarly incorporates an intensive program of monitoring that is typically facilitated by state medical societies (physician assistance programs).

Essential to the Rush and Talbott programs is an intensive day (and at Rush, also an evening) program combined with the availability of recovery residences. Patients live nearby and participate in the day or evening hospital mode of treatment. Total abstinence from all mood-altering, addictive substances is the primary goal, along with establishing nonchemical coping skills necessary to secure quality sobriety. Early in both programs, patients are placed in recovery residences which are structured as "surrogate families." It is here they learn to trust, share, communicate and play, while their nuclear families are given the option to partake in intensive family programs.

PHASE I
EVALUATION TO DETERMINE INPATIENT OR OUTPATIENT TREATMENT

A comprehensive evaluation determines the need for treatment and level of care that will best suit a patient's situation. One focus of this evaluation, conducted by a multidisciplinary team, is to assess the need for inpatient treatment. If such treatment is needed for detoxification and stabilization, the option is available to do so on a limited or extended basis. In the initial interview, the person's needs and how to meet them are determined. The following issues are considered when determining whether inpatient placement is necessary, and if needed, the duration of stay that may be necessary before starting our Phase II:

1. The need for detoxification.

2. The need for acute medical or psychiatric/neurologic stabilization (particularly for patients for whom a dual diagnosis is suspected) . Patients who are actively suicidal or homicidal, or have a history of such behavior, are at risk.

3. Identify patients who are in extreme denial, or who are hostile or resistant to therapy.

4. Identify patients who have an overwhelming compulsion to use a given substance.

PHASE II
INTENSIVE DAY/EVENING HOSPITAL

This phase can follow the evaluation and/or inpatient experience (Phase I) or can be instituted immediately if the criteria listed above are not present and there are no other needs for inpatient treatment. Some health professionals are placed directly in Phase II if, for instance, they have had previous treatment. At this point, there is an individualized approach to treatment planning for the health care professional. This phase involves either day or evening outpatient settings that may include involvement in an independent living community (ILC), which typically involves patients living in monitored apartment settings provided by the treatment program. Each apartment represents a surrogate family environment (Talbott, 1984).

There are four levels of care available in Phase II (Table 2-2):

Table 2.2

Placement Criteria for Phase II Treatment Level of Care Options

Clinical Circumstances	Care Options
Early in disease (stable work and home situation)	Intensive evening program
Early in disease (unstable home situation or need for bonding)	Intensive evening program with ILC
Progressed in disease (high-risk work situation)	Intensive day hospital
Progressed in disease (unstable home situation or need for bonding)	Intensive day hospital with ILC

1. Intensive evening program (patient lives at home and works during the day).

2. Intensive evening program and ILC (patient lives in a residence setting and works during the day).

3. Intensive day program (patient lives at home and may work evening hours).

4. Intensive day program and ILC (patient lives in supervised residence setting and is not working, but involved in a full-time residential outpatient experience).

Intensive outpatient treatment is not only cost-effective (Fink et al., 1985) but also challenges the patient's increasing expectations and discourages the dependence and regression often seen in inpatient settings (Savitz & Kolodner, 1977). Phasing patients into this setting following inpatient stabilization has proven effective historically (McCrady, Longabaugh, Fink, Robert, Beattie, & Ruggierri-Authalet, 1986) and certainly allows multiple levels of care and extended treatment at a reduced cost. Whether the health care professional needs the intensive day or evening program and whether or not he or she will be attending either of these programs while living in the ILC must be determined. The following factors determine where patients need to be placed during their Phase II program.

These modifications are specific for regional patients:

1. *Progression of Disease Process.* The majority of health care professionals are encouraged to attend the day program while living in the residence. Those who may be early in their disease and unable or unwilling to spend time away from their job can be considered for the intensive evening program, assuming (among other factors) that there is no risk to patient care or themselves.

2. *Practice Situation.* It is not unusual for health care professionals to be extremely reluctant to give up their practice for a number of different reasons (e.g., finances, poor coverage, fear of loss of position). If there appears to be no risk to the health care professional or his or her patients, a probationary period in the evening program can be initiated. If more structure is needed, the patient is, at least in part, invested in treatment so that recommendations are more readily followed.

3. *Risk Factors.* This is a major category that will determine the individualized treatment plan for the health care professional. Accountability is a major issue when determining whether or not time away from the job is necessary (as outlined above). Again, one of the major considerations is whether or not the individual poses a risk to patient care or themselves (Angres & Busch, 1989). Comorbidity and relationship and/or occupational discord can increase the need for more structured, longer term, treatment experience.

The majority of impaired professionals at Rush do their Phase II in the intensive day program, which meets 5 days a week from approximately 9:00 A.M. to 5:00 P.M., and averages 4 to 6 weeks in duration. Most live in an ILC, while a few commute from home. The combination of the intensive day program and living in the ILC is typically the optimal situation for treatment. Living in the residence, the patient becomes part of the independent community while dealing with issues involving, among other things, denial and learning about the disease process in the intensive day program community (Angres & Benson, 1985). In some cases, we have the flexibility within Phase II to begin using the day residential setting away from the work situation for a period of time. These patients can then graduate into the evening program, return to work, and gradually phase into the aftercare setting.

The Rush program has the flexibility of placing some regional health care professionals in the evening setting inPhase II. This involves a minimum of 6 to 8 weeks, 4 nights a week (averaging $3^1/2$ hours each night), while working throughout the day. These patients tend to be in an early stage of the disease and well motivated, or are patients who have had previous treatment with some success but have relapsed. The evening population may include those who are unable or refuse to leave work, but, in our estimation, pose no substantial risk to patient care or to their own well-being or family system. With these patients, there is a trial period in the evening program for 1 to 2 weeks to determine whether they can benefit from this type of treatment and graduate into Phase III. There are typically enough healthcare professionals in the evening program so that peer grouping can be accomplished.

The health care professionals in the evening program are encouraged to become part of the residence or ILC setting. Typically, there is an apartment solely for the evening program and occupied by many of its participants. This provides a good deal of socialization, increased structure, and contact with the program for those individuals who are remaining at work while in treatment.

At this phase, patients begin their experience in the Caduceus groups that meet on a weekly basis and continue through Phase

III and aftercare, as in the Talbott program. Caduceus clubs or groups represent support groups for physicians. They have a 12-step orientation and can be a bridge to AA. A strong emphasis on AA and sponsorship is recommended throughout treatment, aftercare, and indefinitely. Treatment also includes a group for significant others, that also meets on a weekly basis in addition to the general family program.

PHASE III
MIRROR-IMAGE PLACEMENT

Phase III involves placement in the mirror-image component of therapy. At Rush, this phase has the health care professional remaining in a patient role but taking on some responsibilities at the treatment center. These may include assisting in the urine-monitoring process or orientation of new patients, as well as sitting in on some staffings — all while remaining involved in their treatment setting, but in a senior patient capacity. This is a requirement for all participants whether or not they have gone through Phase I, and no matter how they have done their Phase II program (day or evening, with or without residence).

The placement experience can be modified based on individual patient needs. This mirror-image phase allows for a transitional period with continued confrontation of denial and support of accountability combined with recovery in a structured setting. Placement traditionally occurs in the day or evening or in participating inpatient settings in the area. The placement experience generally involves a 4-week minimum commitment whether in the day or evening program. This is on a full-time basis for most of our health care professionals, and on a part-time basis for the evening patients. The second 4 weeks may consist of a transitional period that further prepares the patients for return to work and community. For example, here they would spend 3 days or nights in a placement setting and 2 or 3 days a week in their work situation. This allows for a gradual return to the work process, maximizing reentry and internalization of coping skills. The average length of stay in Phase III is 4 weeks (the average length of stay in Phase II is 4 to 6 weeks). This gives us an approximate average of 10 weeks of treatment for the health care professional, which, again, may or may not follow inpatient detoxification or treatment. Mirror image as well as the recovery residences are based upon the teaching of humility without humiliation.

In the Talbott program, the mirror-image placement phase requires involvement in one of several off-campus sites. The patient remains in the ILC, but typically obtains a temporary permit in the state of Georgia and works in some capacity at a treatment center (e.g., county-based programs). The patient continues to participate in the independent community, including house groups for the ILC and biweekly Caduceus groups. The length of stay at the Talbott Recovery Campus tends to average 13 weeks.

This phase allows the patient to experience the risk of being a caretaker who also has recovery-oriented needs. Excessive hours at work, perfectionism, and obtaining an inordinate amount of self-esteem from the workplace are constant risks (see Chapter 4) . Additionally, excessive focus on others' needs can undermine self-observation and attending to one's own needs. Finally, the patients in this phase have an opportunity to see themselves as they were only weeks before as they view the newer patient population they are dealing with. This mirroring has benefits in motivating the newer patients as well as reinforcing the dangers of denial and resistance for the patients who are further along in treatment. Phase III in both the Talbott and Rush programs offers the opportunity to confront and process the issues identified above. Both programs consider this phase a critical part of the treatment.

PHASE IV
EXTENDED AFTERCARE
TREATMENT AND MONITORING

Phase IV is a minimum of 20 months of intensive aftercare that follows treatment for all our health care professionals. The aftercare is very regimented, utilizing detailed signed contracts, and required for all our patients, despite the various modifications in treatment they may have experienced during primary phases. The primary aftercare includes weekly monitoring groups, bimonthly meetings with their physician, random urine monitoring (Shore, 1987), and availability of Caduceus AA groups (Martin, 1984). We also provide groups for significant others and encourage their attendance at open Caduceus AA meetings. Participation in 12-step recovery groups and strong sponsorship are critical parts of long-term recovery and an expectation for all patients. There are also 20 months of weekly support and monitoring groups for significant others.

The minimum 20-month aftercare for health care professionals is established with a signed contract. Attendance is a priority in the monitoring process (Canavan, 1984). The participants are expected to attend aftercare, and only absences approved by staff are accepted. After one unapproved absence from an aftercare meeting, a warning letter is sent stating that another absence will result in an administrative discharge from the aftercare program. The urine monitoring system averages two random urine tests a month, although weekly or more frequent random urine tests are often required; this continues throughout the 20-month period. Missed urine tests are considered positive, and all positive urine test results are dealt with on an individual basis by the treatment team.

THE INDEPENDENT COMMUNITY
WITHIN A RESIDENTIAL SETTING

This model involves a highly effective milieu. We see chemical dependency as a disease that disrupts all aspects of a patient's life.

The primary result on the psyche is regression, ultimately through isolation. Recovery, in a large part, then depends on attaining maturity through fellowship. This is best accomplished, in our estimation, through a "tough love" approach, in which optimal frustration through confrontation occurs in a supportive, loving environment. The ILC setting provides a surrogate family in recovery, and issues that arise in the real world are processed within the intensive group experience. Nonchemical coping skills are learned in a setting that allows integration into the larger society (Rosenthal, 1984). The Rush program averages 60% of professionals who usually maintain a high level of motivation with many resources still intact, setting the tone for a confronting environment where peer expectations are high for all patients. Coercion (e.g., licensure issues prior to admission), often an issue in treatment, can be a positive tool in this setting (Deitch & Zweben, 1984). The ideal relationship, as in the Rush and Talbott programs, is for the Physician's Health Committees (individual programs for recovery of physicians and can also be called Wellness, Health or Impaired Physician Committees) and the licensing boards to work in close cooperation.

The small-group process is a key treatment modality within the larger community. Each patient is assigned a primary counselor who works individually with him or her, develops a treatment plan, and, in conjunction with the family therapist, engages the family in treatment, also leading the patients' small group. The program has an average of four groups in the day and three groups in the evening. Some groups are educational and others provide experiential workshops to enhance nonchemical coping skills. However, the process groups, which often work with specific assignments, are a critical element of treatment. Another integral part of the treatment is the spiritual component, not to be confused with any religious affiliation.

ADJUNCTIVE TREATMENTS

Aggressive treatment of comorbidity is critical in assuring the highest possible recovery rates as well as supporting overall wellness (see Chapter 10). Additionally, the use of some antagonists may be beneficial as adjuncts in the treatment of chemical dependency. In particular, naltrexone is clinically beneficial because of its ability to block the reinforcing effects of alcohol and opiates. Naltrexone has been a routine adjunct for anesthesiologists who are addicted to opiates (e.g., fentanyl). Currently, the role of naltrexone is being expanded to adjunctive treatment of alcohol-dependent patients in selected cases as well (O'Malley, Jaffe, Chang, Schottenfield, Meyer, & Rounsaville, 1992). Disulfiram (Antabuse) may also be used in special cases.

APPLICATION TO OTHER HIGH-ACCOUNTABILITY INDIVIDUALS

In our experience, a number of nonhealth care professionals fall into the high-accountability category and do very well in these programs along with health care professionals. In the Rush program, clergy share a good many of the problems discussed earlier for health care professionals, including increased denial and difficulty with self-observation. Also, executives, educators, and attorneys can often bond in an important way in this type of milieu.

Another group of licensed, highly accountable individuals include pilots, with whom Rush and Talbott have had good success in terms of establishing peer support and longterm follow-up that is highly structured and monitored. Clearly, these professionals have several character factors in common with health care professionals, including the common bond of high accountability in their professional activities. Generally, the clergy go through phases II and III (placement phase), whereas pilots and other nonhealth-care professionals are committed to completing Phase II only. Airline pilots and clergy, along with all health care professionals, are mandated to the extended 20-month minimum aftercare program. Interestingly, mirror-image placement has been very beneficial for selected non-health care professionals.

RESEARCH

Controlled, large-scale evaluation studies have shown that abstinence-based treatment methods are indeed effective (Miller & Hoffmann, 1995). This is true not only for the general population but also for health care professionals in particular. Several studies have demonstrated outstanding recovery rates among physicians with appropriate treatment and monitoring. The benefits of long-term treatment for health care professionals was noted in a study of 120 impaired physicians (Smith & Smith, 1991). This study demonstrated that with extended treatment and appropriate monitoring, 85% had extended periods of sobriety. Another study reported a 9-year follow-up of physicians treated for chemical dependency in New Jersey (Reading, 1992). This outcome study demonstrated recovery rates above 83%. Similar studies have been done by the Rush program as well as the Talbott program. The preliminary findings are discussed below.

ILLINOIS STUDY

The Illinois study involved 278 professionals, including physicians (n = 101), who successfully completed the program and entered into an aftercare contract (Table 2-3). Because the physician sample was the largest subgroup of professionals studied, we will provide a more detailed description of their demographic characteristics, drugs of choice, prior treatment, program involvement, and outcome.

Data collection for this study started in April 1985, when the first professionals began their aftercare (the program was established in December 1984). All patients entered into a written aftercare contract that mandated attendance at weekly, professionally facilitated monitoring groups with random urine screens, and interval sessions with their primary physician (i.e., Phase IV). The data were collected predominately from clinical observations (face-to-face sessions) and urine screening to confirm abstinence.

For patients who completed the 20-month aftercare, face-to-face contact continued in most cases, and interviews were conducted by phone or letter from the remaining patients who did not follow up in person. Third-party confirmation from primary physicians or sponsors regarding the status of patients unavailable for continued face-to-face contact was also obtained.

Table 2-3.

Occupation and Relapse Status of Treated Professionals

Occupational Category	No. Treated	No. Relapsed[1]
Physician	101	18
Nurse	70	6
Clergy	29	3
Pharmacist	14	4
Attorney	14	3
Dentist	13	4
Airline pilot	11	2
Educator	10	2
Counselor	6	0
Administrator	3	0
Medical technician	2	0
Psychologist	1	0
Chiropractor	1	1
Podiatrist	1	0
Veterinarian	1	0
Speech pathologist	1	0

[1]Relapse occurred in 18% of physicians and 14% of nonphysicians. $X^2 = 0.42$, df = 1, p = 0.52. The Illinois study involved patients from both the S.A.F.E. program and Parkside program. The current program is Rush Behavioral Health which is affiliated with Rush—Presbyterian—St. Luke's Medical Center, Chicago, Illinois.

A "favorable outcome" in our study was defined as (1) continuous, uninterrupted abstinence from all mood-altering, addicting chemicals, and (2) involvement in all aftercare expectations. This is a more stringent favorable outcome requirement than that established in other similar studies (Morse, Martin, Swenson, & Niven, 1984), in which some degree of relapse was accepted. However, we concur that some relapses can be therapeutic and can be converted into long-term sobriety, as indicated by our results in this area. In both the Rush and Talbott programs a distinction is made between some relapses (often called "slips"), which do not interrupt the continuum, versus a true treatment failure relapse that results in adverse or lethal consequences.

Of the 278 professionals we studied, 43 (15%) are known to have relapsed. As shown in Table 2-3, the proportions of physicians and nonphysicians who relapsed were similar ($x^2 = 0.27$, df = 1, p = .0.60). Of the 101 physicians, 18 (18%) relapsed. Of these, proportionately more were surgeons and anesthesiologists and fewer were in general medicine ($x^2 = 13.45$, df = 6, p < .04).

Relapsing and nonrelapsing patients are further compared in Tables 2-4 and 2-5. Table 2-4 indicates that the modal physician-patient in this treatment sample was a male, middle-aged (interquartile range, 34 to 46 years), married, general medicine practitioner, who was alcohol dependent. Relapsing and nonrelapsing patients did not differ in terms of age, gender, or marital status, although no woman relapsed. Alcohol and opiates were the two most commonly reported drugs of first choice. Considering all specified "drugs of choice," alcohol (60%) and opiates (44%) were the most frequently used, followed by tranquilizers (23%), and cocaine (18%). Oral ingestion was the primary route of administration, and 16% were intravenous drug users. Fewer than one-half of the patients had prior treatment for addictive disorders. Regarding the distribution of medical practices among the program participants, the American Medical Association indicates that 3.5% of U.S. physicians are anesthesiologists, whereas their representation in our sample was 11%.

Forty-six percent of the patients were dependent on more than one drug (34 were dependent on two drugs, and 12 were dependent on three). Altogether, 43 of these patients used alcohol (n = 14), opiates (n = 14), or both (n = 15). Eighteen (90%)

of the 20 patients who used tranquilizers also had used opiates (n = 8), alcohol (n = 7), or both (n = 3). Thirteen (93%) of the 14 who acknowledged being dependent on at least one other drug besides cocaine mentioned alcohol, opiates, or tranquilizers as their coaddictive substance.

Table 2-4.

Pretreatment Characteristics of Relapsing and Nonrelapsing Physicians

Characteristic	Total (%) (N = 101)	Relapsers (%) (N = 18)	Nonrelapsers (%) (N = 83)	P Value
Gender				NS
Male	92 (91)	18 (100)	74 (89)	
Female	9 (9)	0	9 (11)	
Age (years)	40.7 ± 9.5	40.5 -± 9.3	40.8 ± 9.6	NS
Range	25-67			
Marital status				NS
Married	68 (67)	12 (67)	56 (67)	
Divorced	12 (12)	1 (6)	11 (13)	
Widowed	1(1)	1 (6)	0	
Single	20 (20)	4 (22)	16 (7)	
Practice				.04
Medicine	44 (44)	2 (11)	42 (51)	
Surgery	23 (23)	8 (44)	15 (18)	
Anesthesiology	11 (11)	4 (22)	7 (8)	
Psychiatry	8 (8)	2 (11)	6 (7)	
Radiology	4 (4)	1 (6)	3 (4)	
Pathology	1 (1)	0	1(1)	
Trainee'	10 (10)	1 (6)	9 (11)	
Primary drug				NS
Alcohol	42 (42)	6 (33)	36 (43)	
Marijuana	3 (3)	0	3 (4)	
Tranquilizers	6 (6)	1 (6)	5 (6)	
Amphetamines	3 (3)	2 (11)	1 (1)	
Cocaine	10 (10)	3 (17)	7 (8)	
Opiates	36 (36)	6 (33)	30 (36)	
Fentanyl	1 (1)	0	I (1)	
Route of administration				NS
Oral	69 (68)	10 (56)	59 (71)	
Intranasal	13 (13)	4 (22)	9 (11)	
Intramuscular	3 (3)	1 (6)	2 (2)	
Intravenous	16 (16)	3 (17)	13 (16)	

Continued

Any comorbid psychiatric diagnosis[*]	46	(46)	13	(72)	33	(40)	0.02
Mood disorder	23	(23)	7	(39)	16	(19)	NW
Narcissistic Personality disorder	15	(15)	8	(44)	7	(8)	0.01g
Other personality disorder	11	(11)	4	(22)	7	(8)	NS[*]
Prior treatment	41	(41)	11	(61)	30	(36)	.09

° Comparison between relapsers and nonrelapsers.

°Includes general internal medicComparests subspecialties, family practice, emergency medicine, neurology, and pediatrics.

' Includes general surgery and its subspecialties, obstetrics-gynecology, urology, ophthalmology, and otorhinolaryngology.

°Includes medical students and residents.

'Includes Axis I and Axis II *DSM-III* or *DSM-III-R* diagnoscs. Patients could hOtherre than one diagnosis.

ICompares mood disorder versus no mood disorder among the 46 patients with a comorbid diagnosis (excludes patients without a comorbid psychiatric disorder).

g Compares narcissistic personality disorder versus no such disorder among the 46 patients with a comorbid diagnosis (excludes patients without a comorbid psychiatric disorder).

'' Other personality disorders, excluding narcissistic personality disorder.

The relapsing and nonrelapsing groups did not differ in their reported drug of first choice, route of administration, or percentage reporting more than one addictive drug (relapsers, 50%; nonrelapsers, 45%). However, as compared with nonrelapsers, relapsers identified stimulating types of drugs as their primary drug of choice proportionately more often than sedating types of drugs (relapsers, 28%; nonrelapsers, 10%; $p = 0.05$, Fisher's Exact Test [2-tailed]). There was a trend for a higher proportion of relapsing patients to have been in treatment previously (61% vs. 36%, $X^2 = 2.86$, $df = 1$, $p = 0.09$), but none of the relapsers had more than one prior treatment experience. In contrast, 13 (43%) of the 30 nonrelapsers who had previous addictive disorder treatmValued at least two therapeutic trials.

All psychiatric diagnoses were made using the *Diagnostic and Statistical Manual of Mental Disorders* edition available at the time (either DSM-III or DSM-III-R; APA, 1980, 1987) and were based on clinical interviews. Almost one-half (n = 46) of the patients in our sample had a comorbid psychiatric disorder, 14 (30%) of whom had two diagnoses in addition to a substance use disorder. Twenty-three (50%) of the patients with comorbid psychopathology had mood disorders, and 15 (33%) had narcissistic personality disorder (NPD). Six had both a mood disorder and NPD. Eleven (24%) of the 46 had other personality disorders.

Comorbid psychiatric disorders were more prevalent among relapsers than nonrelapsers (x^2 = 5.04, df = 1, p = 0.02), attributable mainly to a threefold higher percentage of relapsers with NPD (62% versus 21%; p = 0.01, Fisher's Exact Test [2-tailed]). The proportion of relapsers and nonrelapsers who had comorbid mood disorders or other personality disorders was not significantly different. Five of the 6 patients with both a mood disorder and NPD had relapsed.

Table 2-5.

Treatment Components for Relapsing and Nonrelapsing Physicians

Characteristic	Total (%) (N = 101)		Relapsers (%) (N = 18)		Nonrelapsers (%) (N = 83)		PValue
Program type							NS
Day	68		11	(61)	57	(69)	
Evening	33	(33)	7	(39)	26	(31)	
Living in residences	80	(79)	15	(83)	65	(78)	NS
Significant other involved in programming	69		10	(56)	59	(71)	NS
Family program	57	(56)	10	(56)	47	(57)	NS
12-Step program	52	(51)	9	(50)	43	(52)	NS

Table 2-5 shows how many physicians were involved in the core programmatic treatment components. Two-thirds entered the day treatment program, and one-third entered the evening treatment program. Of the total group, 79% participated in one of these programs while living in the nearby rehabilitation residences described earlier. The significant others of almost 70% of the patients were involved in the program. Among them, the significant others of 56% of the patients participated in the family portion of the program, and those of 51% of the patients were in the 12-step recovery program. The significant others of 40% of the patients were involved in both.

Neither program type (day versus evening) nor living in residences seemed to affect relapse rates. These data suggest that for an appropriately selected population, an evening program can be as effective as a day program with regard to abstinence rates. Although the differences between the relapse and nonrelapse groups were not statistically significant, involvement of significant others in the family portion of the program or in the 12-step recovery program was most significant for the subgroup who were able to surmount their relapse.

Only 9 (9%) patients were lost to follow-up. However, 8 of the 9 had relapsed, a highly significant proportion compared with nonrelapsing patients ($x^2 = 28.95$, df = 1, p < 0.000005). In this group, either a significant other support system was nonexistent or their support systems were not involved in their recovery. Of the relapsers lost to follow-up, 62.5% had no significant other involvement, compared with 30% of the relapsers not lost to follow-up and 29% of the nonrelapsers. While not a statistically significant finding due to the small numbers of patients in the two relapser subgroups, this is important information for treatment planning and program development. Relapsing patients who are lost to follow-up are considered to be an at-risk group, susceptible to a deteriorating course.

Table 2-6.

Parkside Follow-up Study, 1984-1990

	Abstinent (%)'		Relapsed (%)°	
No. years in extended monitoring				
1	0		12	(16)
2	0		3	(4)
3	15	(19)	0	
4	11	(14)	1	(1)
5	16	(21)	0	
6	7	(9)	0	
7	12	(16)	0	
Total number of patients	61	(79)	16	(21)

'Percentages based on all 77 patients.

We also examined recovery rates in a cohort of 77 patients who had entered the program, then known as Park-side, between 1984 and 1990, and who had successfully completed this primary program and entered into the extended monitoring program. Table 2-6 shows the distribution of this group of patients in terms of their length of sobriety and when relapse occurred during this 7-year period. Of the patients who completed treatment and committed to aftercare, 61 (79%) maintained abstinence for periods of 3 to 7 years. The highest risk for relapse occurred within the first year of follow-up (N = 12). Relapse rates decreased as time in recovery increased. Three additional relapses occurred during the second year, and only 1 relapse (in the fourth year) was recorded thereafter. Furthermore, 9 (56%) of the 16 patients in the relapse group had only limited "slips" and subsequently had 2 or more years of abstinence; the remaining 7 patients (44%) who relapsed were lost to follow-up.

GEORGIA STUDIES

More than a decade ago, a study of Talbott's program was reported, noting a distribution of specialty practices among physicians that was similar to that in the Illinois study (Porter & Smoot, 1996). Likewise, the primary drugs of choice were comparable with those reported in the Illinois study (alcohol, followed by opiates). Furthermore, 65.6% of the participants in the Georgia program had prior substance abuse treatment, compared with 41% of the Illinois sample.

Between 1975 and 1995, 100 consecutive physicians who entered a continuing care contract with Georgia's Impaired Physicians Program were included in an outcome study (Gallegos, Lubin, Bowers, Blevins, Talbott, & Wilson, 1992). Interestingly, this independent study of a regional population of almost the exact size as that studied in Illinois had nearly identical demographic data and very similar outcomes.

Of the 100 physicians in the Georgia study, 77 had maintained complete documentable abstinence from all mood-altering, addicting substances since the initiation of their continuing care contract. Twenty-two of the physicians had a documented relapse, and 1 was lost to follow-up. All but 4 physicians in the relapse group had at least 2 years of continued sobriety since their relapse. Of note, in the total sample of 100, 2 patients had partial treatment and 2 refused treatment after their 96-hour assessment. These 4 individuals, as opposed to the others who had completed an extended-treatment experience in the Georgia program, had relapsed within 12 months after signing their aftercare agreement. Thus, the outcomes of these two independent studies are extremely similar.

With regard to the relapse dynamics of the Georgia group, the physicians who had relapsed within the first year of signing the aftercare contract were more likely not to believe in the disease precept and felt that they did not need the help that was recommended to them. Those who had relapsed after the second year frequently had family and emotional issues that seemed to trigger the relapse behavior.

All physicians who relapsed stated that they had stopped working in a recovery program prior to the relapse. They had either stopped going to meetings altogether or went infrequently.

As in the Illinois study, the majority of patients (11) relapsed in the first year after completion of treatment. The second highest number of relapses (4) was observed in the second year, with a major tapering of relapses thereafter.

Although the Georgia study did not report any statistically significant differences between the relapse and nonrelapse groups in respect to pretreatment or treatment variables, it did not study comorbid psychiatric illness. The Georgia study did, however, emphasize interviews to determine patients' perceptions as to why they relapsed. Whereas the Georgia study determined that a majority of their relapses seemed to result from problems with recognizing the disease and accepting help, and to a lesser extent from family and lesser stresses, the Illinois study demonstrated a high rate of character disorders in the relapse group. Further comparative studies may demonstrate that there indeed is a correlation between character pathology and interference with the ability to accept one's disease and to accept help. This would constitute a pretreatment and treatment variable that may negatively influence outcome.

It is interesting to note that in all of these studies, relapse rates actually represent a lower risk than the overall physician impairment projections often indicate. Listed below are the data of the Georgia studies.

CHARACTERISTICS OF PHYSICIANS TREATED IN GEORGIA PROGRAM, 1975-1995

For the 20-year period from 1975 to 1995, the Georgia Program has records in their database for 2,429 physicians who presented for treatment (all did not complete treatment). Pretreatment characteristics described for the Georgia Program are presented below in Table 2-7 (Porter & Smoot, 1996).

The major difference between the Illinois and Georgia studies is the amount of previous treatments; 65.6% of the Georgia group as compared to 41% of the Illinois group.

Table 2-7.

Pretreatment Characteristics of Relapsing and Nonrelapsing

Physicians: Georgia Program

Characteristics	Total (%)
Gender	
Male	92.8
Female	7.2
Age (years ± SD)	
Male	44 ± 10.6
Female	41 ± 10.2
Race	
Caucasian	95.4
African-American	2.6
Other	2.0
Marital Status	
Married	62.7
Separated	5.8
Divorced	15.8
Widowed	1.7
Single	11.3
Unknown	2.7
Practice	
Medicine'	38.2
Surgery"	18.8
Anesthesiology	12.3
Psychiatry	6.8
All Others	23.9
Primary Drug	
Alcohol	46.7
Amphetamines	3.4
Cocaine	6.9
Opioids	30.4
All Others	12.6
Prior treatment (inpatient)'	
No inpatient treatment	34.4
One previous treatment	30.8

Two previous treatments	18.6
Three previous treatments	9.8
Four or more previous treatments	6.4

Includes internal medicine, general practice, family practice, and emergency medicine. [b]

Includes surgery and obstetrics-gynecology.

N = 2007 (422 missing observations)

FOLLOW-UP STUDY OF THE 100 GEORGIA PHYSICIANS

Gallegos et al. (1992) investigated 100 consecutive Georgia program physicians who entered into a continuing care contract with the Georgia Impaired Physicians Program. All but six completed all phases of the program. All had a primary diagnosis of chemical dependence and 16 had a concurrent psychiatric diagnosis. In terms of descriptive characteristics, this group of physicians was similar to those described in Table 2-7. Their continuing care contract specified that they undergo frequent, randomized, unscheduled urine drug screens, have a primary care physician (a physician who serves as a recovery mentor while assessing progress in their sponsee's recovery).

Each agreed to attend a minimum of five AA or NA meetings per week, and to attend one recovering physician's meeting per week. Many of these individuals also received recommendations for individual, marital, and/or family therapy. Those who had a comorbid psychiatric illness contracted to continue treatment with a personal psychiatrist and take appropriate medications that were prescribed. Each individual was given the opportunity to create their own spiritual program, physical fitness, and leisure schedule. There were monthly follow-up meetings to review the physician-patient 's progress in recovery. Spouses and significant others were also encouraged to attend these meetings. Reports from many sources allowed the Continuing Care Services Program to evaluate an individual's recovery on an ongoing basis.

Seventy-seven (77%) physician-patients from the study group had maintained complete, documentable abstinence from all mood-altering substances since the initiation of their continuing care contract. All of these individuals have successfully completed their continuing care contracts. One of the 77 died in the seventh year of recovery due to sudden cardiovascular causes. One (1%) patient was lost to follow-up. Of the remaining 75, all are practicing medicine currently except the three (3) who have retired.

Twenty-two (22%) physician-patients have experienced a documented relapse. Eighteen of these have undergone another treatment for their chemical dependence. Of those who relapsed, one died during his relapse. All but four (13 of 17; 76%) of the remaining physicians in the relapse group currently have at least 2 years of continuous sobriety since their relapse. Of those who relapsed and are alive, all but 3 are currently practicing medicine; 2 are retired. Only one of the physicians within the relapse group has been involved in a pattern of continuous, chronic, relapsing behavior since the initiation of relapse. This individual is not practicing medicine.

Eleven (11%) physician-patients relapsed in the first year after completion of treatment. Four (4%) relapsed in the second year. Approximately 68% (15 of 22) of all those who relapsed, did so before completing their 2-year continuing care contract. Two patients relapsed in their third year. The incidence of relapse appears to taper off after the third year in the population studied. Only one person relapsed in years 4, 5, 6, 7, and 8 of their recovery. At the end of the study, no person had relapsed in their ninth or tenth year of recovery.

ADDICTION TREATMENT OUTCOMES: A SEVEN-YEAR FOLLOW-UP STUDY

Twenty-one percent of the physician-patients included in the aforementioned Illinois study relapsed following treatment. In this similar Georgia study, 21% relapsed. The other findings were also comparable.

In the Georgia study (Porter, Talbott, & Irons, 1994), all of the physicians (N = 191) who presented themselves for chemical dependence treatment or assessment at the Georgia program in 1986 were identified and information was obtained from charts and continuing care records. Of these, 46 were assessment only, and 35 did not complete treatment, i.e., left against medical advice (AMA), were administratively discharged, or transferred to a more intensive level of care. Therefore, the 110 physicians who completed the full treatment program comprise the group that was investigated.

- The mean age at admission was 43.17 with a standard deviation of 10.92. The ages ranged from 26 to 74. The median age was 42.

- Of the 110, 102 were male.

- Of the 110, 107 were Caucasian, 3 were African-American.

- 102 were allopathic medical doctors, 8 were doctors of osteopathy.

- The 3 most prevalent medical specialties were: internal medicine (n = 22), anesthesiology (n = 20), and general and family practice (n = 19). These findings are consistent with previous studies.

- Of the 110, 64 had previous treatments.

- Only 33 reported using a single drug or alcohol only.

- The 4 drugs most frequently reported as drugs of choice were: alcohol (n = 59), cocaine (n = 11), fentanyl (n = 10), meperdine (n = 9).

- Sixty-four (58%) of the physicians reported alcohol and drug addiction, 31 (28%) reported alcohol only, and 15 (14%) reported drugs only.

- Sixty-two reported "No medical licensure problem at the time of admission." The remainder (n = 48) had some type of licensure problem.

The 110 physician-patients above were mailed letters requesting their participation in this study. Fifty-two agreed to participate, two refused, four had died, and eight did not respond to our request; 44 letters were returned by the post office. Questionnaires were mailed to those who agreed to participate or did not refuse. Forty-six valid questionnaires were returned. The results of this mailing are listed below. (Note: The results of this study are very similar to previous studies.)

RELAPSE INCIDENTS

There were 36 who reported no relapse and 10 who reported one or more relapses. Only one of the 10 was not in recovery at the time of follow-up, although he was on methadone maintenance. Of the remaining 9, only one had been abstinent for less than 2 years and the remaining 8 averaged over 4 years abstinence; all but one were re-treated in a formal program.

According to specialty area, the relapse group consisted of four internal medicine specialists, two anesthesiologists, two emergency room specialists, a dermatologist, and a psychiatrist. By drug of choice, four were alcohol users, two were Percodan users, and one each of cocaine, codeine, Dilaudid, and fentanyl. A demographic comparison of the relapse group (R) (n = 10) with those who reported no relapse (NR) (n = 36) on selected variables shows that the relapse group was younger (45 ± 11 years versus 37 ± 7 years; t = 8.03. df = 44, $p < 0.01$). All 10 of the (R) group were Caucasian and male; 88% of the (R) group had previous chemical dependence treatment, and 53% of the (NR) group had previous chemical dependence treatment. Sixty-seven percent of the (NR) group and 44% of the (R) group listed alcohol as their primary drug of choice. Only one from the (R) group claimed alcohol only, while 30% from the (NR) group did so.

THE RELAPSING PHYSICIAN: WHEN SHORT-TERM TREATMENT FAILS

Talbott and Porter (1994) conducted a study to explore variables that contribute to the successful treatment of alcohol and drug addicted physicians with a history of relapse following short-term treatment. In order to accomplish this task, two samples of addicted physicians were studied. One sample (group A) included physicians who had received short-term treatment (less than 6 weeks) and subsequently relapsed and were then in treatment at Talbott Recovery Campus. The second sample (group B) were physicians who had received short-term treatment, then relapsed, and then successfully completed long-term treatment (3 months or more) at Talbott Recovery Campus.

These two groups of addicted physicians with a history of relapse following short-term treatment both completed questionnaires. The primary purpose of these surveys was to identify "differences that make a difference" between short-and long-term chemical dependence treatment. With group A, the researchers were looking for their subjects retrospective explanations regarding why their previous treatments were unsuccessful. With group **B,** the same information was surveyed, and additionally why long-term treatment was effective for them as compared to previous short-term treatment(s).

Group A were physicians in treatment in 1994 following a chemical relapse; group **B** were physicians who were attending alumni visits held in 1994. Group **B** had returned to work as physicians (mean = 9.6 months, standard deviation = 5.2 months). Of the 117 respondents, 67% had one previous treatment, 9% had two previous treatments, and 24% had three or more previous treatments.

Their average age was 42.92 years (standard deviation = 8.2, range = 32 - 68); 108 were males; 106 were Caucasian, 8 were African-American, and 3 were Asian-American. Their primary practices were internal medicine, 25%; family or general practice, 18%; neurology, 3%; orthopedic surgery, 4%; obstetrics-gynecology 5%; radiology, 6%; and anesthesiology, 24%; 15% listed "other" practice specialties (Talbott & Porter, 1994). Their drugs of choice are shown in Table 2-8.

THE RESULTS

The items included in the surveys were based on the anecdotal experiences of senior staff from listening to many "relapse autopsies." Also, there were several opportunities for respondents to explain treatment failures and successes in their own words. There were a total of 567 classifiable responses to six open-ended questions. A clear pattern developed. The factors by frequency are shown in Table 2-9. Most of the respondents (n = 70) were sober less than 6 months following their previous short-term treatment.

Table 2-8.

Drugs of Choice for 117 Physicians in the Georgia Relapse Survey

	1st Choice (n = 117)	2nd Choice (n = 77)	3rd Choice (n = 31)
Alcohol	43	32	11
Opiates/Morphine	32	21	9
Fentanyl	16	8	0
Cocaine	16	1	3
Benzodiazepines	8	13	3
THC	0	2	4
Process addictions	2	0	1

From a review of the literature, Blondell (1993) reports that treatment outcomes are generally considered to be more favorable for impaired physicians than for the general public. However, he continues, there is no body of evidence that provides substantial support for differential treatment decisions.

Table 2-9.

Factors Contributing to Successful Treatment Outcomes

Factors	Number of Respondents
1. The opportunity to be in treatment with professional peers	122
2. Sufficient time to internalize recovery principles	74
3. Emphasis on 12-step recovery philosophy	67
4. Attention to my personal problems	39
5. Having a comprehensive aftercare plan	35
6. Receiving personalized feedback and useful confrontation	25
7. Learning to accept structure and discipline	18
8. Personal readiness	16
9. Living in a therapeutic community	13
10. Having an opportunity to develop a personal spiritual program	13
11. Assistance with family problems	10

Anecdotally, and from several published reports, it appears that recovering physicians report a wide variety of successful interventions that resulted in their eventual recovery from drug and alcohol addiction. All physicians do not require long-term treatment. However, since 1976, more than 5,000 health professionals have been treated at the Georgia program and approximately 63% of them had received previous treatment.

SUMMARY

Our experience at both the Rush and Talbott programs supports the benefit of specialized treatment for most chemically dependent professionals in health care and other fields. Extended treatment and long-term monitoring clearly are elements helpful in dealing with the issues of accountability, denial, and accessibility of drugs. Careful evaluation of the disease process and patient-care risk factors can allow for some health care professional patients to have a modified treatment plan (e.g., a trial in an evening setting versus an extended experience away from work). It is apparent that specialized treatment, along with family support and involvement, state medical society involvement, contingency contracts, and aggressive treatment of psychiatric issues and other addictions, contributes to very high recovery rates (80% after 2 or more years). It also contributes to a rapid return to sobriety after relapse for more than half of those who relapse. Our research suggests some additional trends:

1. Relapse is not related to gender, age, marital status, prior treatment, or evening versus day programs in the Illinois study. However, significant other involvement and a concomitant psychiatric diagnosis (especially narcissistic personality disorder) appear to have some impact on subsequent recovery for the physician who relapses.

2. Relapse is most likely to occur in the first year of sobriety for those health care professionals who complete specialized treatment and commit to extended aftercare. More than one-half of the relapse group have limited setbacks followed by two or more years of abstinence.

3. Relapse represents the inability or unwillingness to accept chemical dependency as a disease and/or acknowledge the need for help. Also, family dysfunction, other addictions, and problems in coping with stress were major factors in those who relapsed later in sobriety (i.e., after the first year).

3

Intervention with Physicians and Other Health Care Professionals

A ppproximately one-third of all physicians who enter a formal treatment program had had an intervention that precipitated their admission (Talbott, Gallegos, Wilson, & Porter, 1987). Intervention is often necessary because of the unique and massive denial system that keeps these individuals from reaching out for help (Gallegos, Veit, Wilson, Porter, & Talbott, 1988). Physicians are highlighted, but this specific intervention process can be applied to all health care professionals.

During training, physicians are reminded again and again that they were carefully selected; they are taught to feel unique. They are trained to prescribe drugs and are experienced in handling medications. They are the final decision makers in patient care and consequently develop a sense of control.

Because of this specialized training, many people believe that physicians should know better than to abuse substances or become chemically dependent. Consequently, shame, embarrassment, fear, and guilt fuel the fires of denial in physicians and other health professionals (Talbott & Martin, 1986).

Many researchers have been interested in the sequence in which the capacity of the physician to work, love, and play is damaged by drugs or alcohol. Detection of chemically dependent professionals is often delayed by their ability to protect job performance at the expense of every other dimension of their lives.

Clinical studies suggest that the order in which injury occurs is family, community, finances, spiritual and emotional health, physical health, and finally job performance (Gallegos et al., 1988). The phenomenon of family, neighbors, and friends becoming involved in an exhausting conspiracy that enables the alcoholic to maintain the appearance of normal job functioning is both common and tragic.

THE INTERVENTION PROCESS

Appreciating that intervention is a necessity, the Georgia program adopted a set of cardinal intervention rules. Modified by experience and time, they still serve as the basis for interventions in Georgia (Talbott & Gallegos, 1990).

1. The intervention is conducted by a team consisting of at least two leaders. These leaders need to be identified by officials from the state medical society's impaired physicians program.

2. Interveners are taught the philosophy that intervention is caring and should not be considered punitive.

3. It is necessary to allow adequate time to accumulate and verify data and identify the confrontation team.

4. The holistic support system — family, employer-employees, friends, church, legal, and financial advisors — needs to be identified to serve as a pool from which the intervention team will be selected.

5. Practice sessions on two to three occasions will be required to allow intervention team members to rehearse and know their roles.

6. The goals and objectives of the intervention team must be clearly defined by everyone.

7. Specific assessment or treatment plans need to be formulated, preferably for immediate implementation.

8. The intervention leaders and the impaired health professional should not have any personal or dependent professional relationships.

9. The denial defenses and response to the intervention by the patient should be anticipated and discussed by the intervention team.

10. Site and time of the intervention need to be carefully selected.

11. The intervention should have no time constraints and should allow for return visits.

Several components of the Impaired Health Professional Intervention Program deserve emphasis (Talbott, 1982).

First, although education for the intervention team is a relatively simple task, the attitudes of individuals who receive this education are critical to the success of an intervention. In recent years, it has been increasingly productive to investigate the role of members of the intervention team who are adult children of alcoholics. These individuals may complicate the process of intervention by their attitudes, and at a subliminal level, they inadvertently may even sabotage the intervention.

Adult children of alcoholics live with secrets and may have learned at an early age that life is safer if they don't trust and don't rock the boat. Intervention is a foreign concept to adult children of alcoholics. It also may represent potential danger because of the resultant anger and hostility that might be directed toward them during the course of the intervention. It breaks down the denial system which has protected them in the past.

Second, health care professionals generally do not relate to one another in the form of confrontation, even if it is done in a caring manner. This approach is reserved for patients. Physicians are slowly attempting to break the conspiracy of silence that perpetuates unhealthy behavior in colleagues. However, the intervention process continues to be a risk most professionals would rather avoid.

Third, the intervention technique of utilizing a team must be explained by the leaders, and the roles of all members of the intervention team must be defined. It may be necessary for the leaders to eliminate some team members who cannot or will not be constructive.

Fourth, and particularly important, is rehearsal. Time must be provided to allow all intervention members to practice their individual roles. This can defuse the denial or hostility that a team member may exhibit.

Fifth, selection of team members is based on the total support system of the individual health care professional. When possible, this support system should consist of family members (including children), peers, persons with professional authority over the individual, members of the clergy, friends, administrators, and officials from the medical, nursing, dental, pharmacy, or counseling societies.

It must be understood by all of the individuals involved in the intervention that this event is usually one of the most profound emotional shocks that the alcoholic or substance-abusing health care professional will suffer. The process should not be hurried.

The hour and location of the intervention is an important consideration. Individualized, repeated, return visits must be both anticipated and practiced to answer questions, further the process, and allay fears and misconceptions. It is critical to appreciate the seriousness of the interventions' emotional impact in order to anticipate and prevent a possible suicide attempt or bodily harm by accident or trauma. Tragically, these possibilities are not uncommon, particularly in impaired health care professionals. Thus, the health care professional should not be left alone after the intervention.

WHY INTERVENTIONS FAIL

Of the hundreds of interventions in which the authors have participated, some immediate failures have occurred. It is important to emphasize, however, that what is initially a failure may plant the seed for later success.

In our experience, interventions may fail for seven reasons (Talbott, 1982):

1. Poor preparation, including lack of information, use of rumors or innuendoes, poor selection of intervention team members, or lack of rehearsal.

2. Peers, partners, and individuals in professional authority were not involved, so no "professional clout" was imposed during the intervention.

3. Support systems were not adequately identified or involved, and critical people, such as the spouse, children, parents, or partners were excluded from the intervention.

4. There was not enough time provided for the intervention, and the intervention was never repeated.

5. Family members, peers, and other team members became enablers who sabotaged the intervention. They should be identified and excluded from the intervention process.

6. Disease education for the interveners was not adequately presented or accepted, so the attitudes and behaviors of the interveners were punitive, hostile, and uncaring.

Selection of the intervention site and time were not appropriate; i.e., it was done in the evening or at a time when the impaired health care professional was chemically dulled.

To provide an example, a typical intervention failure occurred with a structured visit to a surgeon practicing in a rural town with two family physicians. The surgeon was documented to have severe alcohol problems that encroached on his office and hospital medical practice. Without adequate homework, his two family practice partners were not fully interviewed and prepared for the intervention.

In this rural town, 70 to 80% of the hospital census depended on this group and, in particular, on the surgeon. The partners were approached, as was the hospital administrator, who realized that his hospital census and financial security would be compromised by this surgeon's absence during treatment. The three individuals, after hasty consultation, assumed a highly defensive and enabling role for their "stressed out but obviously not alcoholic surgeon." They blocked all attempts at intervention.

It was not until 2 1/2 years later that a successful intervention was achieved with assistance from the state medical society and the medical licensing board, following a serious surgical complication at the hospital.

Retrospective analysis of data relative to intervention supports the notion that careful strategic planning and implementation of an assessment are necessary (Talbott & Gallegos, 1990). Once the intervention has been completed, the physician-patient should be taken immediately to the treatment and assessment center. The patient must receive a clear message that he or she must get help now.

PREDICTING SUCCESS

Annually, more than 100 interventions are performed primarily or secondarily by the Georgia program. Approximately one-fourth of these end with the patient refusing to enter into either treatment or assessment (Talbott & Gallegos, 1990).

Which cases are most likely to have a successful outcome? When job jeopardy, serious family dysfunction, and legal or licensing problems face physicians, they are usually very motivated to enter treatment and follow the intervention team's instructions. Negative outcomes of intervention are often experienced in cases of retired or semiretired older physicians who dodge the intervention by abandoning their careers; or individuals with a comorbid (or premorbid) psychiatric condition that makes them hostile or combative and unable to grasp the significance of the intervention because of paranoia or agitation.

Frequently, these individuals need more than just chemical dependency treatment. Intervention failures from these two complicating factors account for 16% of the total intervention failures seen by our group. Following the cardinal intervention rules has an impact on the success of interventions.

Dr. X was a physician using mood-altering drugs and alcohol to self-medicate. The problem began as legitimate back pain, but over the years he became chemically dependent. His spouse was acutely aware of his dependency, which was exhibited by his volatile moods, disturbed sleep patterns, isolation, and an increase in somatic complaints. She was also observing his tardiness and missed days at work. She read a newspaper article about chemical dependency among physicians and kept the phone number in her purse for 9 months. After a particularly violent argument with her husband, she called the number to report his chemical abuse.

She felt angry and vengeful, but later regretted the decision. She fantasized a loss of income, his forthcoming anger, and others' reactions to their problem. An advocate from the state medical society carefully convinced her to prepare for an intervention. This was accomplished after some planning and rehearsal. The physician surprisingly responded with relief and entered treatment that week. He never irrevocably damaged his license or his job, and the family was encouraged to heal with him in the treatment process. He is currently recovering from drug and alcohol abuse and practices medicine with an intact family system.

With effective intervention, successful treatment and recovery are possible for the impaired health care professional suffering from substance abuse or the disease of chemical dependence. It can also positively affect others in relationships with that individual.

SUMMARY

Intervention is often the first step in recovery from the disease of chemical dependency. It is a sensitive area because it involves a process foreign to most health care professionals. Therefore, it is important that professional input be elicited, and the intervention be planned and rehearsed. Feelings of shame and fear often jeopardize the implementation of an intervention. Family members, friends, and colleagues must also seek support and education during this time.

Here are some final guidelines:

1. Interventions should not be done by one person, particularly not by a family member, but by a team.

2. It is necessary to obtain the help and expertise of others, such as representatives from a health professional advocacy committee (e.g., state or hospital impaired physicians committees) or treatment center intervention teams.

3. Colleagues, administrators, and family members involved in the intervention process also need support. This includes education about chemical dependency (literature, lectures, etc.), 12-step support groups (Al-Anon, CODA, Families Anonymous, or significant other groups offered by state medical societies and treatment programs) , or qualified therapists recommended by treatment programs and state medical societies.

4. Collect, document, and evaluate as much data as you can.

5. Presentation of facts at the time of intervention must be strictly factual. Rumors, innuendoes, and gossip must be avoided.

4

Alcohol and Drug Addicted Health Professionals in the Clinical Setting

Impaired health care professionals within a hospital or clinical setting present a number of unique problems that transcend the usual issues encountered in the diseases of chemical dependency and psychiatric illness. Review of our data and experience reveals four distinct groups of impaired health care professionals in hospital or clinical settings. These include physicians, nurses, pharmacists, and hospital administrators and other support personnel including LPNs, medical technicians, orderlies, and ward staff. While there are similarities among health care professionals, each group presents a different set of problems.

PHYSICIANS

Typically, the hospital is the last place the disease of chemical dependency manifests itself. From the inception of medical training, the physician has been taught that the workplace is sacred. While family, personal health, community, and spiritual, social, and leisure life may become seriously disrupted or even destroyed, the hospital setting will remain protected or relatively undisturbed. Additionally, as mentioned in Chapter 3, identification of the impaired physician is difficult because the dynamics of denial are deeply embedded in these individuals. Often their support systems involve a codependency feeding into the denial. Identification is further complicated by the fact that these individuals are only reluctantly identified by their colleagues. Only during the past decade have the national and state impaired physicians programs broken the conspiracy of silence. The authors recognize that many physicians in the clinical setting have two families, their nuclear family and their professional family. Managed health care has recently pushed the independent office practice into a hospital owned or clinic setting. The personnel supporting the physician indeed become a second, professional family. Many of the dynamics displayed at home intrude into the professional family and vice versa.

Experience has taught us that the impaired physician will display two sets of signs and symptoms that should alert people to the fact that he or she is having problems with substance abuse and is in danger of immediately moving into the disease state. The first set of signs and symptoms comprises the following:

1. Chaotic personal and professional life-style.

2. Poorly explained accidents or injuries.

3. Family and marital discord, often repeated crises at home.

4. Long sleeves and tinted glasses inappropriate in a professional setting (to hide tell-tale signs of substance abuse).

5. Deterioration in personal appearance.

6. Significant weight loss or gain accompanied by sensitivity and hostility when identified.

7. Increased use of perfume, cologne, or breath fresheners.

8. Resumption of tobacco use.

9. Legal problems.

10. Spending sprees, gambling, and risky investments.

11. Increasing medical problems, accidents, or other symptoms requiring medication.

Studies have shown that a combination of these signs constitutes a pattern demonstrating substance abuse; the physician should seriously reconsider the use of any mood-altering drugs and should seek immediate counseling and assessment. Once the biogenetic wall has been crossed and the disease of chemical dependence is present, a second cluster of disease signs and symptoms will be seen:

1. Decrease in performance as related to proficiency and productivity.

2. Deterioration of the quality of record keeping and handwriting.

3. Failure to keep on schedule — late to work in the morning or after lunch, often accompanied by midnight rounds.

4. Failure to follow patients appropriately and consistently.

5. Failure to make appropriate consultations or referrals.

6. Altercations with patients, peers, and fellow health professionals.

7. Poorly explained complications and misdiagnosis.

8. Change in prescribing habits, with an inordinate emphasis on pain, anxiety, and insomnia.

9. Inappropriate or inconsistent telephone interactions.

10. Change in type and quality of controlled substances kept in the office or requested from pharmaceutical representatives.

11. Deterioration in relationships with associates.

An administrator is almost always among the first to become officially aware of disease in the physician. Investigating the validity of a problem in the physician, we have found that the clinical staff and security staff are almost always aware of the problem. When the facts and the hospital gossip reach hospital administration, action needs to be taken. It becomes apparent that intervention is necessary.

Intervention for the impaired physician may be accomplished within the clinical setting if a physician's health committee has been activated, or can be performed by the local or a state medical society impaired physicians committee. Because of the malignant denial of the physician, it is almost always necessary to accomplish an intervention before he or she will come in for treatment.

Over the past decade, a number of progressive hospitals and clinics have incorporated impaired physicians programs or physicians health families into their bylaws so that individuals and committees selected for interventions will be professionally and legally protected. Additionally, this allows the hospital to obtain urine samples for drug screens for cause. This is agreed to when the physicians apply for hospital procedures. A model program of this type has been developed by Northside Hospital in Atlanta and Hinsdale Hospital in Hinsdale, Illinois. However, many hospitals have not yet implemented these programs, which make it necessary for the hospital to seek assistance from the local or state impaired physician committee for intervention.

In both the Talbott and the Rush programs, interventions are no longer directed toward immediate lengthy treatment, but are structured for 96-hour assessments. These assessments dictate that the physician be carefully evaluated by medical staff, a psychiatrist, a neuropsychologist using sophisticated neuropsychological testing, an addiction medicine specialist team, and a family therapist. Only then can appropriate diagnosis and treatment recommendations be made. Such recommendations are relayed back to the administrator, chief of staff, and executive committee. In the Illinois program, the multidisciplinary assessment program is directed by a forensic psychiatrist. These evaluations also involve general fitness for duty for health care and other professionals. It extends the assessment beyond chemical dependency and psychiatric disorders.

In recent years, such interventions and subsequent assessments have been utilized not only for health professionals suspected of substance abuse, but also for those with behavioral problems. These behavioral problems include temper tantrums, involving throwing surgical instruments, berating nurses, or speaking inappropriately with patients. Other inappropriate behavior such as unethical sexual interaction with others is also addressed. Because of cultural and legal issues, aberrant behavior that may have been tolerated during the 1970s and 1980s is not tolerated today. Early intervention and assessments are now mandatory for health care professionals with abnormal or unacceptable behavior.

Once the identification, intervention, and assessment of the impaired physician is accomplished, treatment can proceed. Criteria for various forms of treatment (i.e., inpatient or outpatient) have been established by the American Society of Addiction in Medicine identified as *Patient Placement Criteria* (Hoffmann, Halikas, & Mee-Lee, 1996). Additionally, experience in the Talbott and Rush programs has confirmed that certain elements must be present if treatment is to be successful. These include:

1. <u>Staff</u> well trained to treat physicians.

2. Significant number of other physicians in treatment (i.e., peer treatment collegiality).

3. Physician treatment model that is sophisticated and not time-limited.

4. Relationship to the state impaired physicians programs and the state licensing board.

Critical to the treatment is adequate monitoring and aftercare. When the physician returns to the clinical setting, the administration, staff, and patients must be assured of safety. Therefore, a tight monitoring program, supervised by the hospital, and prepared by the treatment facility is a requirement not only for patient safety but also for the recovering physician's benefit. Even if the physician has not gone through a formal treatment program, he or she should go through a 96-hour assessment so that administration can be assured of patient safety and prepare an adequate monitoring and aftercare program. The elements of a quality monitoring program for physicians should include:

1. A written monitoring contract for 5 years (i.e., very exacting monitoring for 2 years and more flexible monitoring for the subsequent 3 years).

2. An *addiction* medicine specialist, who will supervise all of the impaired physician's medical care but not act as the physician's counselor.

3. A *monitoring* physician who will collect body fluids and monitor professional behavior and actions as well as social and familial progress.

4. Reports to the treatment facility and state impaired physicians program from the monitoring physician on a monthly, quarterly, and semiannual basis.

5. Elements within the contract that require regular attendance at AA, individual therapy, and family therapy, if indicated.

If the four elements of identification, intervention, treatment, and reentry monitoring function adequately, physician impairment in the clinical setting can be humanely and therapeutically controlled.

NURSES

Nurses who have alcohol or drug problems generally require treatment and reentry monitoring similar to that for physicians. However, there are apparent differences regarding identification. Both the Talbott and the Rush programs have identified nine commonly encountered signs of substance abuse and impending addiction in nurses:

1. *Severe mood swings.* As the drugs take effect, wide mood swings involving euphoria, anxiety, depression, and anger are present. These are unrelated to situations and events or greatly exaggerated. They often occur after the nurse has been absent for unexplained reasons or has taken prolonged bathroom breaks.

2. *Increased isolation.* This manifests usually as a breakdown in communication with fellow staff workers. Shame, embarrassment, and fear are the bases of this isolation.

3. *Withdrawal from family, friends, and coworkers.* The isolation begins to manifest as the absence from socializing at luncheon meetings, parties, or picnics.

4. *Illegible or sloppy charting.* The impaired nurse's charting will be sloppy, unprofessional, and illegible compared with his or her charting during the predisease period.

5. *Excessive wasting of narcotics.* Needing the narcotics, the impaired nurse self-administers and then records it as a wasting. Substitution with saline or pocketing of the narcotics may be seen upon closer examination of usage. Sedative hypnotics or opioid pills may be substituted in the same fashion.

6. *Frequent medication errors.* These are ways of obtaining a supply of the drug needed by the addicted nurse.

7. *Excessive use of the narcotic room keys.* Guarding the supply is a survival requirement of an addicted nurse. Often she or he will appear on the unit during a day off or outside working hours, for that is where the supply is.

8. *Changes in mental status.* Drug addiction in the nurse will produce acute mental status changes and eventually long-term mental changes. Denial by both the nurses and their coworkers may make these signs more difficult to recognize (i.e., prolonged bathroom breaks).

Frequent disappearance during the shift. It is usually imperative for the opioid-addicted nurse to use parenterally. This will require frequent unexplained absences or long bathroom breaks. A long-sleeve dress or shirt is often worn in hot weather to hide needle marks.

As symptomatic behavior on the unit becomes less subtle, emotional abnormality is readily apparent to peers and nursing supervisors. The depression, excessive emotional outbursts of anger, or apparent anxiety are usually obvious, allowing immediate identification of the problem.

Intervention with the impaired nurse requires that those who intervene be nurses of the same gender. Physicians intervening with nurses are not as effective as peers. Experience has taught us that intervention by non-nurses is much less constructive, as is that by males intervening with females. As with the impaired physician, the support system should be part of the intervention whenever possible. The financial aspects of treatment and reentry, as well as the licensure and job security, have to be considered in an effective intervention.

Treatment and reentry for an impaired nurse are similar to that for the physician. The principles and elements previously described for physicians should be in place when, after treatment, the nurse chooses to come back to service in the clinical setting.

PHARMACISTS

Hospital pharmacists are members of the hospital professional staff who may have an alcohol or drug problem. As is true with nurses, treatment and reentry are in principle the same as that for physicians. Identification is the main difference. Both the Georgia and the Illinois programs have treated a considerable number of pharmacists in their impaired pharmacist group. A list of symptomatic factors has been established to identify the hospital pharmacist suffering from drug abuse or the disease of chemical dependency:

1. *Unexplained and repeated tardiness and absenteeism.* Neither coworkers nor supervisors know where the person is or what he or she is doing during work hours. Long bathroom breaks may be a part of this pattern.

2. *Increased medication errors.* This is not a casual or chance problem. It is usually a deliberate action for guarding or obtaining the supply of drugs.

3. *Drug inventory problems.* As with the above distribution problems, this relates to obtaining drugs for self-medication to satisfy the requirements of the disease or abuse.

4. *Change in work patterns and work effectiveness.* Withdrawal, hangovers, or toxic states from the drugs can produce these changes.

5. *Severe mood swings that produce problems with peers, patients, and supervisors.* These usually manifest as depression, anger, anxiety, or hostility.

6. *Repeated and severe physical, emotional, and situational problems that require medication* by personal prescriptions or self-medication or the inappropriate use of over-the-counter drugs.

7. *Legal problems.* These usually center on community difficulties.

8. *Severe personal, marital or family problems* that begin to encroach on work performance.

9. *Evidence of altered states of consciousness, alcohol on the breath, or traumatic bruises or injuries* (usually late in the disease process).

These signs will begin to cluster, and in late stages of the disease will all be present. Psychiatric illness manifested in behavior is readily apparent, but must be differentiated from drug withdrawal or toxic states from drugs. In hospitals such as the model program at Northside in Atlanta, these signs would be immediately referred to the hospital's Well-Being Committee. A well-being committee is a group of physicians, nurses, or other health care professionals chosen by hospital administration and staff to attend to the problems of their peers, including alcohol and drug abuse as well as other personal matters that may affect the well-being of the professional and the quality of patient care. The committee typically responds in a therapeutic and supportive manner while being sensitive to patient care.

Once intervention for the impaired hospital pharmacist is deemed necessary, as with the physicians and nurses, certain elements must be present for it to be successful:

1. Peers must direct the intervention.

2. The support systems must be present and involved. The state pharmacy advocacy programs and pharmacy boards are ideally involved.

3. The tone of the intervention must be caring, not adversarial, and not time-limited.

4. The possibility of loss of job and licensure has to be explained if the hospital pharmacist will not accept help.

Like physicians and nurses, properly identified impaired hospital pharmacists for whom intervention has been initiated, if adequately treated and placed in a quality monitoring and aftercare program, have an excellent chance for recovery.

ADMINISTRATORS AND OTHER HEALTH SUPPORT PERSONNEL

Both the Talbott and the Rush programs have identified a fourth group of health care professionals prone to substance abuse and addiction, consisting of hospital administrators and other health support personnel. These hospital support personnel include LPNs, nurses aides, orderlies, and counselors. Obviously, physician assistants with drug or alcohol problems need to be dealt with through the primary physician for whom they work. Their intervention requires those physicians to be present and supportive, and can be implemented through the hospital's well-being committee. The LPNs and nurses aides are handled through the nurses' program, while the orderlies and other staff support personnel can be treated through the employees assistance program, which is an integral part of the hospital's well-being committee (as exemplified by the Northside Hospital program in Atlanta).

Both the Talbott and the Rush programs have treated a number of hospital administrators. Administrators possess some unique features because their status is not the same as that of physicians or other hospital support personnel. The most satisfactory results have come about when administrators are treated in the same type of program used for high level executives. From time to time, we have invited them to visit the Caduceus Club (see Chapter 5) to see how impaired physicians, nurses, and pharmacists function in recovery. However, we then place them back in the nonprofessional recovery groups that are aptly termed the real people groups. Because of their positions of authority in the hospital and consequent control over professional staff, their monitoring and aftercare have to be carefully crafted. The well-being committee also monitors the administrators.

Health care professionals from all areas can and do have an excellent recovery rate if the four critical elements — identification, intervention, treatment, and reentry monitoring — are carefully constructed and implemented through a sophisticated and caring hospital well-being committee.

5

Continuing Care and Reentry for Physicians

Continuing care is very important in treating chemical dependency in the health care professional. The period following treatment is a vulnerable time. Our studies suggest that the longer the recovery period, the greater the probability of long-term sobriety (see Chapter 2). Other studies have suggested a similar outcome (Valiant, 1996). The authors' studies have shown that complete rebalance of the neurotransmitter system, along with cessation of withdrawal symptoms, takes much longer than initially postulated. It is not only critical in achieving total abstinence from mood-altering, addicting chemicals (MACS) after the treatment process, but also in providing support and monitoring. In addition to the goal of complete abstinence from MACs, quality of life is an essential aspect of overall sobriety, and strong aftercare programs will help support the health care professional in this aspect as well. In terms of accountability for patient care and overall public safety, aftercare also provides the capacity to verify that abstinence is being maintained. It also allows for early detection of relapse as well as prerelapse elements.

The formal duration of aftercare has often been modified in terms of the various elements involved. Many state medical societies and licensing boards have addressed the issue of duration of aftercare. In general, 2 years of continuing care has been a minimum requirement for most monitoring entities as well as specialized treatment programs for the health care professional. However, to better ensure longterm recovery, as well as to maximize support and ensure public safety, continuing care has often been extended to 5 years, or even longer in some states.

The continuing care settings that exist throughout the country today for the health care professional reflect much of the original Caduceus Club components spearheaded in the early 1970s by Talbott. The Caduceus Clubs are regarded as a bridge toward not an alternative to Alcoholics Anonymous (AA) and other 12-step programs. The basic components of the Caduceus Club involve a commitment to a strong 12-step recovery program such as AA or NA, involvement of the significant other whenever possible, a weekly group meeting, and adjunctive random urine monitoring. As both treatment and continuing care capacities evolved over the last decade, there has been a tendency toward separation of the Caduceus Club concept and formal aftercare in most areas. With the growing sophistication of state medical societies' physician programs that often sponsor or provide aftercare programming, further separation between the Caduceus Club concept and formal aftercare has occurred. Although there are variations on a state-by-state basis, the following components describe basic elements of a strong continuing care program and monitoring system.

REENTRY AND CONTINUING CARE FOR HEALTH PROFESSIONALS

Frequently, when addicted doctors have reached the point in their disease where they must leave their practice for treatment, their professional life is in shambles. Patients, staff, peers, and coworkers are often frightened, confused, and angry. For many, the fear of returning to work is profound. In addition to these relationship issues, there may be real concerns about "Fitness for Duty." Evaluating fitness for work, a service provided by Rush and Talbott programs, is an independent part of the treatment. These evaluations generally cover three interrelated aspects of functioning:

Knowledge and skill. It is important to assess the physician's body of knowledge related to his or her specialty. Remedial education may be needed. Also, questions about dexterity and the use of instruments and devices need to be answered. Frequently, working under the close supervision of an accepted expert may be necessary to make the determination.

Medical/neuropsychological. A thorough physical examination, including blood chemistry workups designed to identify alcohol or substance abuse and other abnormalities, is essential. Comprehensive psychiatric, psychosocial, psychological, and neuropsychological assessments are included. It is not unusual to find that the alcohol addicted physician has incurred neuropsychological impairment to the extent that practice is unsafe until remediation and healing has occurred. Also, there are other physical abnormalities that have been untreated that are identified which need remediation.

Commitment to recovery. When, and if, the diagnosis of addiction has been made and substantiated, it is important to assess the physician—patient's personal commitment to recovery. Also, to assess their available resources to assist in maintaining a recovery program. Commitment to recovery is best determined by behavioral changes. Much of what is looked for is included in the *Sixteen Points* discussed in this chapter under continuing care considerations. Being teachable and following instructions are fundamental in recovery. A goal is to become comfortable in recovery and to bond with other recovering individuals. Patients are encouraged to "stick with the winners." As is true with many chronic diseases, daily attention to the disease process and its remediation are important, to prevent relapses and deterioration.

REENTRY PLANNING

Since a major goal of treatment is to assist recovering alcoholics and addicts to return to their professions and utilize their healing attributes, reentry planning begins at the beginning of treatment. The interactions between their disease and their work are carefully examined. Many have used their medical privileges to obtain their drugs and their workplace was the equivalent of a bar or crack house. These "triggers" need careful attention and neutralization. It is not unusual to have a doctor state that they justified their drug use by rationalizing that they could better deal with the pain and discomfort of others if they first medicated their pain and discomfort. As part of reentry, addicted doctors must reconstruct their personal relationship with mood-altering substances.

Intensive reentry work needs to be part of the treatment. The intensive work is best done in small groups of doctors who are near the end of their treatment. The group setting allows the participants to share their feelings and fears, and work together on problem solving. When at all possible, it is insisted that each doctor preparing for reentry return to their home or office for an extended visit (generally 5 days) where they are able to get a feel for the environment and set up continuing care safeguards. In addition, it is frequently required that a physician or dentist in treatment visit the workplace of a recovering colleague and experience the sights, sounds, and smells of the workplace. It may involve going into an operating room as an observer. Also, this is an excellent opportunity for the physician in treatment to converse with a successfully recovering physician about return to work issues and feelings.

ANESTHESIOLOGISTS

Anesthesiologists are overrepresented (Talbott et al., 1987) among chemically addicted physicians. It is yet to be determined if it is the temptations of anesthesia that cause this phenomenon, or if physicians with addictive predispositions tend to choose this specialty. This will not be addressed here. However, there are those who feel that once anesthesiologists become addicted, they should no longer be allowed to practice anesthesia. The authors do not necessarily agree. If a treated anesthesiologist meets the fitness for work requirements, there are many who can safely return to anesthesiology. The following schematic has been utilized with favorable results:

Anesthesiologists' Return to Practice

Category I (Return Immediately)

1. Accepts and understands the disease.
2. Bonding with AA/NA.
3. Healthy and strong family support.
4. Committed to a 2-year contract of recovery.
5. Balanced life.
6. No presence of psychiatric disease or personality disorder.
7. Good treatment experiences with support from staff members to return to anesthesiology.

Category II (Reassess after 2 years)

1. Relapse occurred but demonstrating recovery.

2. Family members improving, but remain dysfunctional.

3. Involved but not yet bonded with AA/NA.

4. Healthy attraction to anesthesiology.

5. Recovery skills improving.

6. Some denial remains — but continues to work on honesty, open-mindedness, and willingness (HOW).

7. Continued mood swings but no presence of psychiatric disease or personality disorder.

Category III (No return)

1. Prolonged intravenous use.

2. Previous treatment attempts failed; relapses.

3. Disease present and attracted individual to anesthesiology.

4. Severe psychiatric disease or personality disorder.

5. Inability to follow a treatment contract.

6. Poor recovery skills with no bonding in AA/NA.

7. Severe family dysfunction.

GOING BACK TO WORK

In addition to dealing with all the feelings and fears of family and friends, the treated physician must now face office staff, peers, colleagues, competitors, and patients. Often the major questions of the returning physician concern what they will disclose to others about their past, present, and future. Generally we advise them to tell others honestly only what they need to know. Knowing what they need to know requires considerable attention that should be done in professionally led groups prior to leaving treatment. It is important that the returning physicians not make these decisions alone. Frequently, fear, shame, or anger distorts communication, and more harm than good is a potential hazard.

Occasionally, physicians will have key office staff attend family programs at the treatment center. Paying this level of attention to the workplace has proven valuable for all involved. It is not uncommon for the office staff to be the physician's chief enablers. They can also play an important role in relapse prevention when they are adequately informed.

The most diverse group facing the reentering physician appears to be peers and colleagues. They can fall anywhere between extreme support to absolute rejection. Many are anxious to be of assistance, others are judgmental and unforgiving. It seems that untreated adult children of alcoholics can be the most negative. Physician—patients are urged to accept help when it is offered, recognize the fears of others, and learn to depersonalize rejection. An important concept for the returning physician is that they are sick and not bad. Honesty tempered by discretion is the preferred course of action.

It is often a surprise to returning physicians that their patients, as a whole, seem to be the least affected and most accepting of all those they encounter upon return to work. Of course, there are exceptions.

ANTABUSE AND NALTREXONE

While the programs are based on the 12 steps, abstinence and nonchemical coping, two pharmaceutical agents are used in recovery. Disulfiram (Antabuse) is used in very selected cases, where its contraindications are clearly eliminated. Naltrexone for opioid and alcohol users is frequently prescribed for its anticraving properties and can be an effective adjunct in recovery.

CONTINUING CARE MONITORING AND SUPPORT GROUP

This group ideally is professionally facilitated by a mental health professional with appropriate credentials, an understanding of chemical dependency, and, when necessary, overall psychiatric issues as well. The group should function primarily as a monitoring group. In other words, the recovering health care professional can be observed in the group process to determine the strength of his or her recovery program and the areas of actual or potential concern. The group should also, however, provide support as well as an element of insight-oriented psychotherapy. Clearly, there are potential issues regarding trust and the ability for patients to fully disclose. However, with a skilled group therapist, the group members are able to recognize that they can trust in the group while being monitored by the group leader. These groups, like the continuing care process in general, involve an advocacy-driven process. The purpose of the monitoring is not to catch someone in relapse, but to prevent relapse from occurring. When relapse does occur, one must attempt to intervene in such way as to transform that relapse into a learning experience that may be translated into long-term sobriety. However, the group process, like the continuing care process as well, must be based on the recognition that the recovering health care professionals are licensed to provide quality care to the public. The health care professionals must recognize their responsibility not only to their own recovery and their family, but to their patients and the general public as well. A sense of participation in the accountability aspect of recovery is essential. This needs to be an established component of the group conscience. With the recognition of group conscience comes some acceptance of the responsibility that, whether involving relapse or relapse dynamics, there may be consequences in the continuing care setting. For example, if an individual has persistent thoughts of using drugs because they are being unduly exposed to MACs on the job, then this may need to be addressed by significant changes in the workplace or a change of workplace altogether.

The continuing care monitoring and support group should meet on a weekly basis. Attendance must be taken and any absence must be appropriately excused, except in emergency circumstances. Excessive or unexcused absences would be considered a violation of the aftercare agreement. Group participants need to know that elements critical to their recovery and practice are shared with the monitoring entity responsible for their care and advocacy. These groups are often facilitated through specialized treatment programs as done at both Rush and Talbott. In areas where specialized programs do not exist, these groups and the continuing care, in general, typically are facilitated by the state medical society physician assistance programs or the licensing boards.

It is helpful in the continuing care meetings to have a group of 5 to 10 peers that meet on a regular basis. The involvement of the main significant other (MSO), in their own group, is significant in the recovery process for both the patient and the MSO. A 16-point checklist is helpful for group members and the patient when assessing progress and continued effort in recovery.

SIXTEEN POINTS

1. Meetings

2. Sponsor

3. Monitoring

4. Emotional traps (anger, guilt, depression, anxiety, insomnia, etc.)

5. Additions/subtractions to addiction history (secrets)

6. Compulsive behavior (sex, food, nicotine, gambling, theft, spending)

7. Current therapy/ treatment/medications (prescribed, OTC)

8. Relationships (family, spouse, MSO, parents, children, friends)

9. Physical health—exercise program

10. Leisure time-fun

11. Work (professional status, duties, attitudes)

12. Financial status

13. Legal—licensure status

14. Additional training and/or continuing medical education

15. Spiritual program

16. "Soft" part of your recovery program

RANDOM URINE MONITORING

The urine monitoring component of continuing care provides objective evidence of either nonuse or use of MACs. Urine monitoring should be performed on a random basis, an individual typically providing a sample within 12 hours of an initial call. The random urine monitoring component can be facilitated through any number of entities. The primary monitoring entity may be a treatment program, state medical society physician assistance program, a hospital, a group practice, or the monitoring physician. Several of these entities may monitor the recovering health care professional.

In addition to being random (requests for urine coming on a random rather on regularly scheduled bases), these urine samples must be handled in a chain-of-custody system. There must be careful observation with the monitoring individual responsible for making sure that the urine sample ends up directly in the designated laboratory without the possibility of sample altering during or after the process. The urine panel should include testing for all major MACs (Fluharty, 1996). In certain cases (as with anesthesiologists, for example) regular additions to the panel are needed.

The best example is screening for fentanyl or sufentanil. These opiates, along with hydrocodone, typically are not part of initial screens and must be added. Additionally, drugs such as naltrexone, which is taken as an adjunct to reduce craving and block the reinforcing effects of alcohol and opiates, also require a specific request for testing.

The frequency of urine testing depends on each individual case. A typical standard regime is two random urine tests monthly. The randomness of the drug screens, which means it is not anticipatory, is critical in health professionals. The frequency can be weekly, twice weekly, or even more frequently when indicated, thus being varied throughout the course of an individual's aftercare, depending on the need. For example, testing frequency may be high during the first 6 months of recovery, then begin to decrease as more stability in recovery is demonstrated. Increased frequency can also occur during times of stress or general vulnerability to relapse. Urine screening should occur anytime there is undue suspicion of substance use. This can be initiated by any of the monitoring entities, or even by the recovering health care professional him- or herself to demonstrate that substance use is not an issue. A chain of custody for each monitored urine is essential.

A positive urine test result that is documented on thin-layer chromatography must be confirmed by gas chromatography/mass spectrometry. Possible false positive or marginal positive results need to be clinically correlated. Any confirmed positive result must be dealt with in an aggressive fashion. Confrontation of the individual accompanied by further exploration and additional documentation is necessary in cases of tested individuals not admitting drug use in light of positive urine test results. Classical examples of poppy seed ingestion giving false positive opioid results in the urine drug screens have been encountered in the Rush and Talbott programs.

MONITORING PHYSICIAN

The monitoring physician is typically an addiction-oriented physician who takes responsibility for meeting with the recovering health care professional, usually on a quarterly basis but more frequently if needed. The *monitoring* physician is responsible for ensuring compliance with the continuing care contract and recovery program. The *treating* physician is typically the physician who had followed the patient during the active treatment program. The treating physician is identified as the confidant.

During the quarterly visits by the monitoring physician, information should be documented regarding compliance with the continuing care monitoring and support groups, 12-step recovery programs, work and home environment, presence or absence of craving, and overall urine monitoring status. There should be ongoing communication between the monitoring physician and any other entities involved in the monitoring process. This may include the state medical society physician assistance program, hospital-based wellness committee, supervisors, and, if involved, representatives from the licensing boards.

PERSONAL PHYSICIAN

The personal or primary physician is the primary caregiver to the recovering health care professional. This is the physician responsible for the overall health maintenance of the individual. The personal physician should be aware of addiction issues and the health care professional's addiction history. This is particularly important in situations that might require administration of MACS, e.g., surgical procedures and acute or chronic pain situations. The personal physician then has to communicate with the monitoring physician regarding any problem that might arise.

PRACTICE MONITOR

In certain cases where there is considerable concern regarding the health care professional returning to practice, a practice monitor is sometimes assigned. This is an individual who is able to conduct ongoing observation of the recovering health care professional. It may be someone involved in a similar kind of work, who is able to observe professional practice by chart review and periodic random visits to the office or health care setting. The practice monitor should be someone who is familiar with the addictive process and in a similar area of specialty as the individual being monitored.

12-STEP RECOVERY
AND CADUCEUS GROUPS/CLUBS

An integral part of the continuing care plan is 12-step recovery program involvement. This includes either AA or NA involvement with sponsorship. Regularly, the individual agrees contractually to be involved and be active in these support groups. Typically, a minimum of three meetings per week is required. Occasionally there are individuals who consistently resist attending support groups and who may substitute other kinds of support groups acceptable to the monitoring system (e.g., Rational Recovery). Caduceus groups, which usually represent a bridge to 12-step recovery that is specific for health care professionals, are a critical part of recovery. Most areas in the country have some form of Caduceus program available. A minimum of one Caduceus meeting per week is requested. As mentioned earlier, Caduceus clubs are a bridge, not a substitute, for 12-step recovery.

Some Caduceus groups offer additional sessions for significant others of recovering professionals. These are not structured as 12-step meetings, but as supportive-learning groups, and they are optimally led by a qualified family therapist. In the experience of the authors, it is best that these groups be conducted in a confidential manner and that they offer a safe place for significant others to discuss their personal issues and concerns. If the group becomes a means of monitoring the recovering professionals, it not only loses its effectiveness but may also compromise the significant other's safety issues. In the Talbott and Rush programs, these groups are conducted simultaneously with the Caduceus continuing care groups.

RETURN VISITS TO THE TREATMENT FACILITY

At the Talbott and Rush programs, as in other treatment facilities, return to the treatment site for alumni visits are strongly encouraged. Talbott Recovery Campus contractually requires patients and their MSO to return after 90 days, one year, and 2 years. At Rush the visits are voluntary and offered every 3 months. At both Rush and Talbott these visits are 48 hours in length and are scheduled for Monday and Tuesday so the patient is able to attend the Caduceus Group on Tuesday evening. Return visits have been reported as being a positive influence in maintaining a solid program of recovery.

TREATMENT CONTRACTS

The Rush and Talbott programs have experienced the value of treatment contracts. While not useful or valid as legal documents, they are helpful in clarifying expectations of the treatment facility to the patients and their professional affiliations. Listed in Table 5-1 is an example of a Continuing Care Contract employed by the Talbott Recovery Campus.

Table 5-1.

Sample Continuing Care Contract

Discharge Date: Name:

Home Address:

Phone: (H) (W)

1. I agree to participate in Continuing Care for 5 years from my date of discharge.

2. I agree to abstain completely from any mood-changing chemicals except as prescribed by my primary care physician.

3. I agree to follow the terms of my relapse contract (see attached).

4. If I change my address, I agree to notify the Continuing Care Coordinator within 2 weeks after such a move.

5. I will obtain and execute new release of information forms on each yearly anniversary date of my discharge.

6. I will practice my work/profession in the following location: Address: Phone:

7. The following are specific problems regarding my hospital, licensing board, DEA, etc. (include prevailing restriction).

8. I plan to return to work by:

9. I plan to work the following hours per week:

10. I will use as my primary physician:
    Name: Address:
    Phone:

11. I will use as my monitoring professional:
    Name: Address:
    Phone:

12. I agree to random urine/blood monitoring drug screens to be set up by and agree to pay for this urine/blood drug screen.

13. I have asked the following person to be my sponsor and to actively

14. work with me on 8th- and 9th-step issues.
    Name:
    Address:
    Phone:

15. I will initially attend 90 12-step group meetings in 90 days, followed by attending at a frequency of 4 to 7 times per week.

(continued)

Below are the AA/NA meetings available in my area

Day Monday	Type of Meeting	Location	Time
Tuesday			
Wednesday			
Thursday Friday			
Saturday Sunday			

Additional Comments:

16. I agree to attend the following Health Professionals group (e.g., Cadu- ceus Group, if applicable):

    Name:

    Location:

    Contact Person:

    Phone:

17. I agree to attend the following continuing care group, if applicable: Name of Group:

    Time:

    Location:

18. I agree to participate in individual, marriage, or family therapy, if applicable:

    Therapist:

    Time:

    Location:

19. I plan to return for the following continuing care visits (to include Continuing Care Conference and/or Caduceus Retreat):

    a

    b

    c

20. I will continue to develop my spiritual program of action (pages 85-88 *Big Book*) by:

21. I will continue to invest in my family life by:

22. I will continue to develop my leisure time by:

23. I will continue to maintain my physical health by:

24. I plan on assuming responsibility for all expenses connected with my treat- ment, and all previous debts, if applicable, by:

Patient's Signature   Date

Continuing Care Coordinator   Date

6

Relapse and Recovery

Relapse is a characteristic component of the disease of chemical dependence and is defined by us as resumption of the intake of mood-altering drugs or alcohol following a recovery process. Relapse typically occurs unless potentially contributing factors are recognized and addressed (Vaillant, 1980). These trigger mechanisms are believed to be similar for most people suffering from chemical dependence (Talbott & Cooney, 1982), but some aspects seem exacerbated for people in the health care profession (Robinowitz, 1983; Vaillant, 1970; Woolf & Bennett, 1983).

RISKS FOR RELAPSE

The time of greatest risk for relapse is the first 2 years after entering treatment. This, of course, provides the rationale for having extended treatment time followed by a lengthy aftercare period

(Talbott, Holderfield, Shoemaker, & Atkins, 1976). Caduceus aftercare forms a network for interrupting relapse when it does occur and helps health care professionals return quickly to the terms of their aftercare contract.

CHEMICAL DEPENDENCY AS A DISEASE

The fundamental factor believed to precipitate relapse is a failure to understand and accept the precept of chemical dependency as a disease. Clinical experience, research data, and animal-cellular experimentation all have contributed evidence substantiating the belief that chemical dependency is actually a primary psychosocial — biogenetic disease; the term *disease* is not merely a useful theoretical category (see Chapter 1).

Chemical dependency has been shown to exhibit a general but variable symptomatology, to have certain biogenetic and psychosocial components, and to follow a generally predictable course leading, if untreated, to death (Valiant, 1983). That chemical dependency is a disease is axiomatic for all practical purposes. Alcoholism and other drug addictions are considered slight variations of the same disease.

The acceptance of this may be a matter of life or death for people with the disease. If people who are chemically dependent do not accept their condition as a disease, there is no reason for them to abstain from mood-altering drugs and the disease will become active again.

It would seem that physicians, of all people, would readily accept this disorder as a disease; however, it has been our experience that the majority do not. All too often, we have found them to be more resistant than other people to such classification. There are several reasons for their reluctance.

Until very recently, little information on alcoholism and drug addiction was presented during medical training, except for discussion of complications to the various organ systems involved in the last stages of the disease. Historically, little or nothing was taught about the diagnostics or dynamics of the disease. Also, the prevailing thought in our society regarding alcoholism and drug addition is that it is, at best, a matter of poor taste, and at worst, a moral or psychological problem. Physicians are products of their culture and tend to hold beliefs similar to those held by the rest of society.

The variety of symptoms of chemical dependency, which may or may not appear in different combinations in any individual case, also makes it difficult for people to conclude on their own that they are chemically dependent. Even the compulsion to use drugs is not present all the time. Many people can stop using drugs — they just cannot sustain abstinence. Thus, the nature of the disease itself, with its variety of signs and symptoms, contributes to the confusion (Gitlow, 1980) and lack of acceptance of the precept. The disbelief and the fear, disgust, and moral indignation of people in the family (Jackson, 1954) and community who do not understand chemical dependency certainly add to the confusion and discomfort of people who have the disease (Wallace, 1977).

Before Prohibition, American physicians treated alcoholism as a disease, but since Prohibition, the culture has considered chemical dependency a bad habit resulting from immorality or a weak will (Bissell & Jones, 1976). Although chemical dependency is similar to diabetes in some respects, the attitudes regarding relapse in these two diseases are quite different. We have yet to hear emergency room health professionals say to a returning patient, "Not you again, you dirty diabetic!" Yet on several occasions we have heard similar remarks used with a relapsing alcoholic or drug addict.

DENIAL

Denial is another important contributing factor in relapse, while it is almost universally present with the disease. It involves lack of acceptance of the disease on a personal and emotional level rather than on a cognitive level. It involves failure to make the connection between abuse of mood-altering chemicals and the problems that follow. People in denial often continue the same behavior pattern while expecting different results. Denial, as seen in the alcoholic or chemically dependent person, is used as a defense, but is more global in nature than that seen with neurotic persons. The dynamics of denial, while comprising a mosaic of pharmacologic and emotional factors, derive from physical and emotional pain. The physical pain associated with the effect and withdrawal of mood-altering chemicals is coupled with the fear of powerlessness, the need to believe that one possesses self-discipline and thereby can control most aspects of one's life. This combination makes the disease with its compulsion difficult to accept personally.

Most physicians believe that the exercise of self-discipline leads to extensive control of the immediate environment. Acknowledging the disease and surrendering to the treatment and life-style of recovery is difficult for most doctors and impossible for some. The dynamics of holistic denial make it very difficult for impaired physicians to reach out for help, even if they overcome the denial of self-identification as an alcoholic or drug addict (Talbott & Gander, 1975; Tiverski, 1982). Also, they are unlikely to get help if they seek it. In a survey of male alcoholic physicians who had been abstinent for at least 1 year, Bissell and Jones (1976) found that 77.6% of interviewees had sought professional help for alcoholism, but the doctor they had approached did not recognize alcoholism as the problem.

Initially, chemically dependent physicians use denial to deal with the painful dissonance caused by discrepancies between mind and reality (Frolich, 1972). Discrepancies between the way people perceive events and the situational realities form the basis for alienation. One such discrepancy exists between the physician's knowledge of pharmacologic effects of drugs and their lack of personal acceptance of the process of addiction in their own lives. Another is seen between personal experience and knowledge of the results of chemical abuse and their compulsion to use chemicals anyway.

Such a cognitive dissonance, documented extensively by Festinger, leads the health care worker to resolve the conflict or defend against it with mechanisms such as denial (Festinger, 1957). After weeks or months of abstinence, denial may again become potent. Many health care professionals who have been through intensive treatment, including cognitive and experiential learning about the disease of chemical dependency, may still at some stage of recovery seduce themselves into believing that all of these facts and experiences they have learned no longer apply to them. They tell themselves that they can drink or use drugs again and "control it this time." They believe that they have learned enough to drink appropriately; "like everybody else." The disease seems to progress even during abstinence, and many people in relapse do not make it back to treatment before they die (Zuska & Pursch, 1980).

FAMILY ILLNESS

Another factor that contributes to relapse is the family system. The dynamics of the family play a part in the progression of addiction, and these same forces play a part either in recovery or relapse (Finley, 1983). If the family understands and accepts chemical dependency as a disease, and if family members have a program of recovery for themselves, the responsibility for sobriety and spiritual development is appropriately returned to the person who is chemically dependent; the family is then free to give support without ambivalence. This person with the disease, not the family, is responsible for the outcome. If this appropriate assignment of responsibility does not happen, then the same enabling and dysfunctional behavior seen in the progression of chemical dependency recurs and can contribute to continual relapse (Bennett & Woolf, 1983). With continued relapse, there is almost always an individual or individuals who serve in the role of enabler.

DISHONESTY

In many instances, dishonesty is difficult to separate from denial. The dishonesty that occurs is not usually "cash register" dishonesty, but rather emotional variance from the truth. This often manifests in extramarital affairs, questionable business or political deals, social misconduct, and lying about or breaking appointments. Alcoholics Anonymous (AA) recognized this problem early on and stated that there were some unfortunates with the disease who could not recover because they were constitutionally incapable of being honest (Bennett & Woolf, 1983). Impaired health care professionals who have undergone extended specialized treatment have identified honesty as one of the most critical components of their sobriety and recovery, and one of the most difficult qualities to maintain.

LACK OF A SPIRITUAL PROGRAM

Lack of a spiritual program also has been cited frequently by recovering health care professionals as a factor in relapse. The emphasis in recovery is on spirituality, not on a specific religion. The steps in the AA/NA spiritual program consist of acceptance of the disease, surrender to a higher power, work on removing personal character defects, and service to others. The second step of AA states that individuals who recover are those who come to believe that a power greater than themselves can restore them to sane living. Without surrender to this force, alcoholics and drug addicts continue to attempt recovery alone and thus feel in control, isolated, and sick. As a consequence, many of them experience relapse. There are those who do not accept the concept of a higher power, and may benefit from alternative groups such as "Rational Recovery." In the experience of the authors, however, these people appear to struggle in their maintenance of a recovery program.

CROSS-ADDICTION

Cross-addiction persists as a frequent contributor to relapse in impaired physicians and, far too often, to their unintentional death by overdose. Unlike laypeople who believe a doctor's prescription is inviolate, physicians know the pharmacologic effects of the drugs they prescribe. Therefore, they often eschew prescription drugs and resort to over-the-counter drugs, getting into trouble as a result. Many drugs cause unintended effects when combined with other drugs or with alcohol. They also cause unintended results when the tolerance level changes abruptly, as it does in the chemically dependent person. Consequences can be especially destructive if the physician, having identified narcotics as his or her drug of choice, then turns also to other pharmaceuticals, alcohol, or marijuana to seek relief.

STRESS

Stress in the form of job demands, marital or family discord, or emotional crises will often precipitate relapse. Initially, as well as in the early years of recovery, people who are chemically dependent do not have the capability to deal with stress nonchemically. Yet this capability is exactly what they must learn to remain sober. Treatment facilities often teach "non-chemical coping skills" for emotional and situational stress resulting from insomnia, anxiety, sorrow, guilt, and depression or other feelings. Meditation, exercise, and nutrition, and involvement in team activities and sports are taught and encouraged as mechanisms to combat stress.

EMOTIONAL AND PHYSICAL TRAPS

The emotional and physical traps of hunger, anger, loneliness, fatigue, and self-pity have been identified by the recovery community over the years as key factors in relapse. The slogans of "HALT" ("Don't get too Hungry, Angry, Lonely, or Tired") and "PLOM" ("Poor Little Old Me") have been adopted by AA as admonitions to help avoid traps that can lead to relapse. Health care professionals, because of the nature of their work, often delay meeting their basic physical and psychological needs for an extended period of time. This delay can contribute to self-pity as well as to physical and emotional depletion, thereby contributing to thoughts of relapse, and later to the relapse itself.

ISOLATION

Isolation, either in the form of physical isolation from others or staying away from the recovery community and its meetings, can also precipitate relapse. Physical isolation, often caused by the professional's duties, needs to be offset by contacts with family, friends, and the recovery community. When people stay away from meetings, they usually go back to friends and places associated with the days of drinking or drug use, and relapse soon follows. Such associations are particularly attractive and influential during the first few years of recovery. Abstinence from mood-altering chemicals leaves a void which is believed to be biochemical, psychological, and spiritual in nature. That void must be filled with positive feelings associated with people and activities in the present and relationships and events that strengthen sobriety and spiritual development. Otherwise, the person seeks to fill the void with recalled feelings of euphoria associated with chemicals.

CONTROL

Another area of extra difficulty for health care professionals is related to control issues. Most have a high need for achievement and control, and their training has reinforced and refined these characteristics. In their work, health care professionals are accustomed to being in control of themselves and other people around them, both ancillary personnel and patients. They see their major task as eliminating or controlling pain and the disease process. It is, therefore, most difficult for them to give up control and to join others in fully accepting the first step of AA: "we admit we are powerless over alcohol and that our lives have become unmanageable." The honesty expressed in this step, however, is necessary to begin the process of recovery and to maintain it in the face of life crises that occur with everyone, regardless of chemical dependency. Health care professionals must deal with their patients' life crises as well as their own and consequently need a constant reminder of their inability to manage single handedly. A similar group of chemically dependent individuals struggling with control issues includes lawyers, clergy, pilots, and high level executives.

INCREASED VULNERABILITY OF THE HEALTH CARE PROFESSIONAL

The nine factors described above are believed to contribute to relapse in people with chemical dependency. Certain circumstances have been noted which seem to increase the likelihood of relapse for physicians and other health care professionals. Obviously, the chances of becoming cross-addicted are better than average with health care personnel because of the ready access to drugs. The seemingly innocent use of a substance other than one's original drug of choice can lead back to alcohol or to the abuse of other drugs (or a combination of the two). Drugs play an important role in treatment protocol for patients of health care professionals. Also, physicians are known for their preference for self-medication. These conditions contribute to increased vulnerability to chemical abuse, leading to dependency.

OTHER ADDICTIVE BEHAVIORS

Addictive behaviors such as compulsive gambling, overeating, and sexual acting out are common among chemically dependent people. Sometimes this is a substitution phenomenon, other times the substance abuse curtails these compulsions. In either case, these compulsions can become pronounced during recovery from alcoholism or chemical dependency. This, in turn, can lead to problems with shame, guilt, diminished self-esteem, and relapse. Specific treatment tracts have evolved in treatment programs to address these behavioral addictions. Twelve-step groups such as Overeaters Anonymous, Sex Addicts Anonymous, and Gamblers Anonymous can be extremely effective in treating these behaviors.

PREVENTION OF RELAPSE

Knowledge and acceptance of relapse as a major aspect of the disease, along with an attitude of cautious optimism regarding sobriety, form the basis for uninterrupted recovery, one day at a time. Chemically dependent health care professionals who become lax about going to meetings, grandiose and overconfident about their "cure" and complete recovery, and unconvinced of the actual principles of recovery are in serious danger of relapse. Denial, compliance, and grandiosity are major threats to sobriety.

Prevention of relapse begins with the continual awareness of the possibility of this painful and often disastrous complication. The way to prevent relapse is to develop personal spiritual strengths along with nonchemical coping mechanisms for dealing with other environment and accompanying feelings. A person thereby accumulates a reservoir of experiences in the successful use of these mechanisms and can draw on it in times of stress. In addition, he or she develops a network of supportive relationships for giving and getting compassion and help. A blueprint for this kind of development is found in the steps, the philosophy, and the structure of AA and NA. Based on spiritual principles, the steps are concrete actions taken by people in the AA/NA fellowship. They are suggested as ways to enable people to chart their progress on the road to recovery. The philosophy teaches that perfect recovery is not attainable, but progress is. The structure of the AA/NA fellowship stresses democratic participation in the meetings and other activities as well as being of service to others.

The primary characterization of the chronic disease of alcoholism and other drug addictions is the compulsion to alter one's mood through the use of chemicals. With the elimination of this one-dimensional coping technique for all situations, both victims of the disease and their families often fail to take note of the serious possibility of relapse. The resumption of chemical coping following a recovery process is a fairly common occurrence and, although not happily welcomed, must be honestly faced. In no way should confronting this issue before it happens be construed as permission or encouragement for relapse to occur. Rather, dealing with this possibility allows people with the disease and their families to acknowledge their ability to handle the event, gain proper perspective, and use the experience as they would any other in the recovery process. All too often the relapse is precipitated by a trauma, surgical or dental procedure, or by pain, which is self-treated or treated by a physician unknowledgeable in the field of chemical dependency.

Alcoholics Anonymous speaks of "stinking thinking" as the prelude to actual drinking and drug use. A recovering physician echoed the AA/NA philosophy when she said, "I alone can do it, but I cannot do it alone, for isolation and aloneness are the assassins." This chemically dependent physician has admitted to having thought of or planned a relapse before actually consuming the drug. This is true for most alcoholics and drug addicts. It is, therefore, urged that if the desire or compulsion arises, the patient should take the following steps before using a chemical (and certainly if one has already used a chemical). These steps should be included in a "Relapse Contract." An example of one is inserted at the end of this chapter.

1. *Call his or her sponsor.* Every impaired health care professional should have a sponsor in AA or NA, and preferably talk to that sponsor daily for the first 5 months of recovery. The sponsor must be called before a drink is taken.

2. *Go to a meeting* immediately and daily thereafter, or more often if needed, to resolve the conflict over using.

3. *Call AA/NA friends and share honestly with them* either the urge or the incidence of using.

4. *Contact by phone or in person his or her treatment center or primary addiction physician* and discuss the addiction truthfully.

5. *Admit and discuss* in detail at the AA/NA meetings the compulsion or relapse.

6. *Pick up the white chip at a meeting – begin* again with the first step.

7. *Talk with spouse, family, and/or significant other.* Although it may be difficult for them to accept relapse, it is recommended that it be shared.

If impaired health care professionals and their family members are committed to recovery, then they will need to understand and use these guidelines. Families and significant others are advised to do the following:

1. If they are aware of the relapse of a loved one before he or she talks about it, they should call their sponsor in Al-Anon / Nar-Anon and contact person at the treatment center.

2. Go to Al-Anon / Nar-Anon meetings daily; discuss the relapse and their feelings until they have resolved any conflict they have about the situation.

3. Detach from the patient with love and continue their lives.

4. Reinforce their own recovery programs through Al-Anon /Nar-Anon contacts and friends.

5. If a loved one talks of a relapse, listen openly, support the person, and turn the responsibility back over to him or her. With health care providers, it is recommended that a sponsor or advocate be notified by the significant other.

6. If the person does not admit and discuss the relapse, the family member shall follow the advice of his or her sponsor and treatment center as to the possibility of intervention.

If impaired health care personnel and their family members are committed to recovery, they will use the above guidelines as needed and will involve the primary care physician. When informed of a relapse, the primary care physician will assess the situation and make recommendations both to the patient and to the treatment center staff, who may deem it necessary to insist on additional hospitalizations or treatment, or at least immediate and frequent drug screening. Although it is not usually necessary, direct intervention in some cases can be life-saving. In most cases, relapse can be interrupted simply by implementing the guidelines presented above. Members of the support system are contacted to offer support and cooperation to increase the probability of early interruption of the relapse. The pre-relapse signed contracts are invaluable in confronting the denial of the health care professional, family, peers, and other members of their support systems.

INDIVIDUAL DIFFERENCES IN RELAPSE

Components of the disease of chemical dependency and factors of recovery generally are similar for all impaired people.

However, individual differences are present, and their recognition is important in several ways. The drug of choice, route of administration, and extent of medical complications may contribute to a different overall disease pattern. Sex and ethnic background, a well as the life-style and presence of a support system, also may modify the pattern of addiction and response to treatment programs.

Furthermore, people in certain occupational groups have been found to be especially resistant to treatment, such as physicians and other medical personnel. Part of their difficulty in maintaining sobriety lies in their personal and family background, their training, and their drug history. Another part certainly involves the ambiance of their work environment and traditional position in the community. A treatment program must be able to accommodate these individual differences to foster a patient's acceptance of the disease precept and identification with peers. Only then will channels of communication be in place for constructive confrontation and support.

Of course, similar conditions are utilized in AA and NA through self-selection. People in AA/NA choose a home group with which they identify and it becomes their reference group. It provides support as well as confrontation for personal and interpersonal growth.

SUMMARY

Relapse can either be a treatment failure or just another milestone on the road to recovery, depending on the attitudes and interactions of the patient, family, treatment personnel, and other support systems. Relapse is an ever-present possibility, both universal and individual in nature. People recovering from chemical dependency learn which methods work best for them to deal with their life crises and their "dry drunks" in order to ward off a "wet drunk" later on.

The continual process of recovery is the important thing to remember. The following is an anecdotal recovery story.

A pharmacist was discovered to be diverting oral opiates at the workplace. After intervention, she entered a treatment program for chemical dependency. She was compliant with all treatment components except for the recommendation that she not return to retail pharmacy work. She returned to the workplace with an intensive monitoring program, including frequent random urine tests, a naltrexone Caduceus aftercare program, and documented attendance at 12-step meetings. Within 6 months, she had a urine test result positive for opiates. The treatment team confronted her and she admitted using drugs intermittently for 3 weeks. It was recommended that she not return to retail pharmacy work for 1 year, and that she attend 90 meetings in 90 days and 2 weeks of an evening program. She complied and returned to work a year later with significant modifications to the workplace, including strict supervision by a coworker and minimal handling of mood-altering substances. She currently remains in solid recovery.

Finally, here are two lists indicating contributing and preventive factors of relapse.

Factors that contribute to relapse:

1. Denial

2. Family system

3. Dishonesty

4. Lack of a spiritual program

5. Cross addiction

6. Stress

7. Emotional and physical problems

8. Isolation

9. Control

10. Other addictive behaviors

11. Stop attending meetings and practicing the program

Factors that help prevent relapse:

1. Knowledge and acceptance of the disease

2. "One day at a time" attitude

3. Regular attendance at 12-step meetings and the presence of a strong sponsor

4. Development of personal, spiritual, and nonchemical coping skills

5. A network of supportive relationships

6. Attendance at other 12-step recovery groups as appropriate (e.g., Overeaters Anonymous, Gamblers Anonymous, Sex Addicts Anonymous)

7. Involvement of the family members and support systems in recovery.

Below is a relapse contract utilized by the Talbott Recovery System.

RELAPSE CONTRACT

I. I, , should I use any alcohol or other mood-altering drugs, agree to perform the following:

a. Contact my AA/NA sponsor.

b. Attend an AA/NA meeting and pick up a white chip when applicable.

c. Contact my monitoring professional in my area to inform him/her of the relapse.

d. Contact the Director of Continuing Care at Talbott Recovery Campus to inform them of the relapse.

II. I, , as a member of the family or significant other, agree to encourage the patient to contact the monitoring professional to inform him/her of the relapse. I agree to contact my sponsor and home Al-Anon group for additional suggestions. I agree to contact the monitoring professional and the Director of Continuing Care at TRC as outlined above if the patient is unwilling to do so.

III. I, , will complete and return this contract to TRC within thirty days of discharge.

Patient Signature	Date
Family member/ Significant Other	Date
Monitoring professional	Date
Director of Continuing Care Talbott Recovery Campus	Date

7

The Medical Marriage
and Recovery
from Chemical Dependency

t is often stated that marriage is work and we are warned that
the three most common marital problems are about sex, money,
and in-laws. Most of us underestimate the amount of tenacity
involved in living and compromising with another human being
on a daily basis. Physicians and their spouses, in addition to the
problems common in all marriages, face unique problems related
to their personalities and profession. These unique features are
the very problems that are exaggerated in chemically dependent
relationships. First, there are problems in communication that lead
to isolation. Second, there is loss of identity and subsequent low
self-esteem of the spouse. Finally, the need for intimacy, which
differs between partners from the start, disappears completely

with the disease of chemical dependency. This chapter will use case studies to illustrate these problems.

MEETING THE NEEDS OF SELF-ESTEEM

The unique nature of the medical marriage is attributed to two major factors: the demands of practice and the psychological makeup of the physician. According to Gabbard and Menninger (1988), the physician chooses a nurturing mate to override his or her fragile self-esteem, which often is a problem dating back to childhood. Valliant, Sobowale, and McArthur (1972) found physicians, as compared with a control group of nonphysicians, more apt to have suffered from emotionally impoverished childhoods (this is the perception of the physician and not necessarily reality). Physicians choose mates who they believe can provide the nurturance they missed when they were children. However, once they secure the relationship with this mate, they do not totally accept the nurturing. Their self-esteem needs are better fulfilled by colleagues, patients, and the community. This is clear in the following case study.

> Dr. X, a physician who had undergone treatment for chemical dependency and had spent 1.5 years in recovery, relapsed on hydrocodone. He used the drug for approximately 1 week, during which a colleague noticed some changes in his behavior. All of Dr. X's colleagues were well aware of his disease of chemical dependency and were very supportive of his continued recovery. When the colleague noticed the change in the behavior, he telephoned Dr. X's wife and asked if he had relapsed. The wife confronted her husband that evening, but he assured her that he had not relapsed. One week later, Dr. X's urine tested positive for his drug of choice. He was confronted by his physician from the treatment program. Dr. X then admitted using the drug and stated that he wished he had confided in his colleagues earlier. No mention was made of his wife. In

another room, Dr. X's wife stated that she was very em-
pathic and available during the time she confronted her
husband about his drug use, and yet he denied it. She
wondered what was wrong with her and their relationship that made Dr. X unable to trust her and allow her
to nurture him during this stressful time. She had also
been working in a program of recovery for 1.5 years in
Al-Anon and other significant-other groups.

THREAT OF INTIMACY

Dr. X was uncomfortable when his wife attempted to offer her
love and acceptance. He was more interested in the respect and
fellowship of his colleagues. He was able to attain esteem from
their approval without the threat of intimacy that his wife posed.
When intimacy was controlled, as it was with the low level of
intimacy between physician and patient, it was comfortable. It
often becomes difficult for the physician to go beyond this, even in
those relationships that demand more intimacy to be successful.

Of course, this greatly affects the medical marriage. The physician chooses a spouse based on that person's ability to nurture,
and then shuns the very quality that is desired. Communication,
intimacy, and self-esteem are all affected by this contradiction.

PERFECTIONISM

Other personality traits that characterize physicians are
related to compulsiveness. These traits are perfectionism and
excessive dedication to work (Gabbard & Menninger, 1988).
Compulsiveness is a favorable trait when career success is the
focus, but does not fare well in relationships with other people.
The physician is unable to relinquish this trait when interacting
with his or her spouse and family. It is easy to see how the medical family suffers as a result of this, but the physician also suffers

consequences. The most prevalent one is guilt or the painful feeling of regret, as shown in the following case.

> Dr. P was a physician just out of residency. He and his wife had three young children. He had joined a very high-powered group in a competitive climate with other specialists. His wife thought that when he completed residency there would be more time for family life. However, it seemed that Dr. P was away from home more than ever. His wife would complain, and often those complaints erupted into bitter arguments. She resented his profession for taking valuable time away from her and their family life. He, on the other hand, resented his wife for not understanding the demands of his practice. They both attended separate aftercare groups; he for chemical dependency and she in the significant-other group. In these groups, they frequently discussed their feelings and resentments. He felt guilty for being unavailable to his wife and family, but he also felt guilty and anxious if he took time away from practicing medicine. She felt a loss of self-esteem due to his assumed lack of interest in her needs and their marital relationship.

GUILT

The guilt for taking time out for leisure coupled with the guilt of not being a good enough husband or father left Dr. P with a feeling of overwhelming helplessness. His wife was feeling lonely and her self-esteem was low. They both were angry and resentful, blaming the demands of practice for their disharmony. Actually, lack of time for leisure, family, and self, or the demands of practice, is a *symptom* rather than a *source* of marital conflict (Gabbard & Menninger, 1988). It is also a major factor that contributes to the unique nature of the medical marriage.

Gabbard & Menninger (1988) believe that physicians become workaholics to compensate for their perceived emotional impoverishment. They also believe that it is not the demands of practice but the compulsive personality of the physician that causes conflict in the medical marriage. As we see with Dr. P, the guilt of spending too much time away from home only results in more time away. To compensate, the physician needs colleagues and patients to reestablish self-esteem. As mentioned earlier, they can provide mirroring needs without the threat of intimacy. Both spouses suffer from this lack of intimacy.

INTRUSIONS TO INTIMACY

The beeper (pager) and the telephone are related to the demands of practice. They are constant reminders, even when not in use, of the physician's primary responsibilities. Medical families can give numerous examples of these types of intrusions into their personal lives. The following case is an example.

> Dr. A is a psychiatrist with a wife and two preschool children. He is on call every other weekend. One of these weekends, the family attended a picnic and looked forward to a day together. The beeper and portable phone accompanied Dr. A throughout the day. During the day, Dr. A received a page and spent approximately 1 hour speaking intensely and pacing back and forth. Later, Dr. A explained that he had been talking with a depressed patient. The wife felt guilty because she resented the patient for ruining their day. She did not share these feelings with her husband but the resentment persisted.

DELAYING GRATIFICATION

How often have these words been spoken in the medical marriage: "After medical school it will be better. . . . After residency things will change. . . . After the boards we'll be O.K. . When the practice is solid we'll have the time and money. . . "? The phenomenon of postponement or delayed gratification is commonplace in medical marriages. It is also related to the demands of practice, which keep the medical family in a holding pattern. Living for the future takes away the valuable time we have today and prevents spontaneity and enjoyment. It leaves one with the feeling that things can only be good when the physician succeeds in reaching a particular goal, but the goals are endless. Again, it is really not the demands of practice but the physician's compulsion that causes this phenomenon. Many of the traits that make a good physician also create a destructive family life.

The unique factors discussed above are applicable to all physicians and their spouses. Discussions that follow focus on the traditional medical marriage: the physician husband and the nonphysician wife. Some of the points will be universal. Nontraditional physician marriages, however, have unique features. Many of these features will be mentioned in Chapter 8. In contrast, the effects of chemical dependency are not confined to any one group of individuals or type of relationship. Disease does not discriminate in its ravages.

THE MEDICAL MARRIAGE
AND CHEMICAL DEPENDENCY

Let us look at what happens when the physician is chemically dependent. All healthy aspects of the marriage are slowly and insidiously disintegrated until both partners are dysfunctional. The unique features are exaggerated and contribute to the development and perpetuation of the sick, dependent relationship in chemical dependency.

COMMUNICATION DIFFICULTIES

Communication problems in medical marriages arise from differing perceptions of the marriage itself (Gabbard & Henninger,

1988). Generally, women are more able to share their feelings than men. A woman may be aware of this difference before marriage, but hopes that her husband will change. She also may believe that she does not need to hear him express his feelings, as she is so attuned to him that she will figure them out anyway. The following is a case scenario.

> Samantha is a professional nurse in her late twenties who relocated with her physician husband so that he could receive treatment for his chemical dependency and start a new residency. Samantha came to a significant-other group one evening and complained that she was not "being heard" by her spouse. She had been coming to this group for several months and had rarely spoken in the past. This particular evening she asked the group for help in communicating her needs to her husband. The group offered some of their own individual methods of communication; i.e., use of "I" statements and stating feelings, etc. Samantha said she would try these approaches. She returned the following week in tears. She recounted her husband's short, angry responses to her needs and feelings. She identified that her husband was always "quiet," but would "at least listen" to her in the past. In another room, her husband was sharing his feelings with his aftercare group that evening. He stated that he could not meet Samantha's needs and her feelings were too painful for him to listen to. Both were encouraged to continue sharing their feelings in group and to also engage a marriage counselor to assist them in communicating.

The failure to communicate in Samantha's marriage began early in their relationship. He was "quiet," but Samantha felt confident that she could take care of his needs without his input; they were both so busy that there really was not any time to have "deep" conversations. Samantha learned to suppress her feelings so she wouldn't feel out of control. The feelings she denied were the same that are prevalent in many families trying to cope with the disease of chemical dependency: shame, fear, anger, sadness, and loneliness. She learned to blame, threaten, and lie to keep her life manageable, mostly with people outside the marital relationship. In the marriage itself, she shut down and came to accept the lack of intimacy. She denied feelings for so long that she began to believe the delusions. Then she wondered why she felt as if she was going crazy.

In traditional medical marriages, with or without chemical dependency, it has been observed that spouses of physicians typically live with emotionally silent partners and provide unconditional support (Gabbard & Menninger, 1988). The physician expects his emotional needs to be identified and taken care of by the spouse without ever communicating them. To the contrary, the spouse feels frustrated because she cannot identify or fulfill those needs. Feelings of frustration lead to feelings of inadequacy because she blames herself for not being more understanding and supportive. They can live in quiet desperation for years until a crisis occurs — perhaps treatment for chemical dependency or a malpractice suit — then, the marital difficulties become real and insurmountable. Just as with Samantha and her spouse, such couples frequently need professional guidance to help learn how to get in touch with frozen feelings, and to communicate those feelings to each other. Often, in cases of chemical dependency, couples are urged to seek individual therapy separately before entering marital counseling. At the very least, all family members involved with chemical dependency are encouraged to develop their own programs in appropriate 12-step groups.

It is usually difficult for the significant others of alcoholics and addicts to begin their journeys toward self-discovery and recovery. Initially, the spouse of the identified patient is convinced that the problems lie solely with the addict. This belief is expressed by many first-time members of the significant-other groups for impaired health professionals. Often the spouse is asked to verbalize some feelings when they first join the group. It is usually not difficult for them to state feelings, but these feelings usually fall within a very narrow range—sad, mad, and glad. These feelings all relate to another person's behavior. It is frequently a surprise for the significant other to realize that they are unaware of how they truly feel or that people are interested in those feelings. The loss of self that occurs in codependency is most noticeable in these types of group dialogue. This will be discussed in greater detail in Chapter 9.

ISOLATION

When the medical couple, living with the disease of chemical dependency, is unable to communicate their feelings and needs, they learn to live with secrets and shame and slowly begin the journey toward isolation. Think of it as an onion being peeled. The social strata of a family's life are being peeled away as the disease progresses, beginning with the least intimate relationships—social clubs, acquaintances, and professional liaisons. These people are avoided, phone calls are left unanswered, or excuses are given to postpone contact with people. The peeling away of people then moves to more intimate relationships—church or temple friends, coworkers, and neighbors. Finally, the extended family and close friends are peeled away and the sick family unit is all alone to cope with their deadly secrets. The spouse feels more intensely inadequate because she cannot solve the family problems as she did in the past. Communication between marital partners is indirect, unclear, shameful, and blaming. They are alone and lonely in a crisis situation that can only be healed through contact with people who have been through similar crises and professionals who understand the disease.

LOSS OF IDENTITY

The next unique feature of medical marriages with chemical dependency is the gradual loss of identity and subsequent low self-esteem of the nonphysician spouse. The spouse, usually a woman, becomes "Mrs. Daniel Angres," not "Kathy Bettinardi-Angres." The following typical exchange in a support group illustrates this.

Upon entering the significant-other group, individuals are asked to introduce themselves following a brief introduction by experienced group members. The veterans of the group usually begin by stating their names and any other information they feel might help the newcomer know them better and feel welcome to the group. It is always revealing to hear members change these introductions as time goes on. For instance, one member may say, "Hi, I'm Tara and my husband is an ENT surgeon. He was addicted to codeine and alcohol and he's been in recovery for 3 months now. . . . " Another member may say: "Hi, I'm Bunny and I've been coming to this group for 3 months. I am a homemaker with four children. I go to Al-Anon and an individual therapist to work on my recovery. It's not easy but I'm feeling less angry than before. . .

It appears that Tara is still hooked into her husband's identity, whereas Bunny has learned to focus on herself. She may still be struggling with her own identity, but she is taking steps toward self-discovery and recovery. All new members enter the significant-other group focused on their addicted spouse. This is normal for a dysfunctional family. It is much more comfortable to concentrate on the identified patient. Feelings are painful for the significant others, and this outward focus allows them to avoid the pain for awhile. But the anguish will not disappear without being confronted at some point.

Consider the traditional medical marriage without the complication of chemical dependency. The nonphysician spouse, usually a woman, becomes a dependent caretaker in the marriage. She makes many sacrifices for the survival of the family. She is both mother and father to the children much of the time due to her husband's extended hours at work. The verbal or nonverbal message in the marriage is that her job as a homemaker is menial in comparison with the daily life-and-death decisions faced by her physician spouse as illustrated in the following example.

Kristy planned a birthday party for her 4-year-old daughter. The little girl talked about her party with excitement for days. Her physician father promised to be home and share in the festivities. Just as the doorbell rang and the first guest arrived, Dad's beeper went off. Kristy felt that familiar anxiety that arises at the sound of a pager. After a brief phone call, Dad returned looking apprehensive and nervous. He explained to Kristy and their daughter that an emergency required his presence at the hospital. He promised to be home in time to sing "Happy Birthday." Predictably, Kristy's husband did not return until the party was over and their children were long asleep. He shuffled in with bloodstains on his scrubs and a haggard, tired look in his eyes. Kristy was filled with anger and frustration but stifled her feelings. How could she complain about a birthday when someone's life was at stake? She swallowed her anger once again and they silently went through their bedtime routine. He left early the next morning and their feelings were never discussed.

Medical couples have greater dissatisfaction in their marriages compared with nonphysician marriages. The profession comes first in the medical marriage. The spouse often falls into the role of caretaker and becomes dependent on her husband, especially financially. Separation and divorce are often avoided for economic reasons. The nonphysician spouse also becomes dependent on the physician's accolades. In assuming the role of the caretaker, the spouse puts her career and its advancement on hold or second to her husband's career. He holds the most promise for economic and professional gains, so she settles for running things behind the scenes.

Bev Menninger describes the wife's position as "living on the edge of the spotlight." She states that most traditional wives assume from the beginning of the marriage that this is where they will be, and most have chosen to be there.

There are advantages: a comfortable standard of living and the option to stay home and raise their children, but there are risks also. Ms. Menninger lists three risks: (1) diverging activity tracks; (2) responding to a high-achieving husband with a competitive need to do as well or to be the perfect wife, mother, professional, etc.; and (3) living with the M. Deity Syndrome (grandiosity of physicians). The greatest risk, however, is loss of identity and residual feelings of helplessness, resentment, anger, and depression.

THE SPOUSE'S LOW SELF-ESTEEM

When the disease of chemical dependency emerges in the family, the wife's role as caretaker and support system becomes exaggerated. She feels responsible for other people, and even their thoughts and feelings. She feels compelled to solve everyone's problems and feels frustrated and inadequate when she is ineffective. This is such a large task that all of her time is spent ruminating about others. She loses her sense of self, and identity is then derived from what she does for others. Without a sense of self, there can be no self-esteem. Good feelings come only when she is successful in fixing someone else's problems.

The codependent behavior we have described above does not develop overnight. Many times it is a learned behavior from families of origin. It is, however, definitely reinforced in medical marriages and compounded by the disease of chemical dependency.

When an addiction evolves, the medical spouse is somewhat prepared. She has already assumed the role of caretaker, so it feels natural to apply this role to a spouse impaired by chemical dependency. She also feels responsible for him, so she covers up for him, uses drugs or alcohol with him, organizes his chaos, and takes over each of his responsibilities that fall by the wayside.

Many times she does these things without even being aware of the problem, as evidenced in the following example.

Sophie entered the significant-other group for the first time after her physician husband had been confronted by his peers and had just started treatment for chemical dependency. Sophie, on first impression, appeared controlled and defensive. She stated that it was a shock to learn of her husband's disease. They had a "wonderful marriage" and were very close. There were no problems at home and she wondered out loud if this was really happening. Several members asked Sophie to describe her marital relationship. Sophie stated that she and her husband were "dependent on each other." A group member asked Sophie if she and her husband were intimate, if they shared feelings with each other. Sophie said there was no time; her spouse was a resident and spent "90% of his time at the hospital." When he did return home, he mostly slept. Another member asked if she was responsible for the house, children, finances, and social plans? She answered, "Yes." This same member asked, "Aren't you tired?" Sophie hesitated and then responded, "Yes."

Sophie's self-esteem was completely tied into her role as caretaker. It would have been destructive for the group to confront her about her enabling behavior and denial of the disease. Sophie realized these things on her own over time. The process begins with the spouse identifying her own feelings. Even this is difficult for a person who has little sense of self.

When a person sacrifices herself and her identity for the good of others, it is commonly referred to as codependency. Codependency can emerge in other dysfunctional systems or families, but is always earmarked by the overwhelming loss of identity and low self-esteem.

DIFFERING NEEDS FOR INTIMACY

The final feature that distinguishes the medical marriage from other marriages is the differing needs for intimacy between spouses. Gabbard and Menninger state that gender differences are more pronounced in these relationships and are the primary reasons for these differing needs. (This is pertinent in traditional medical marriages only.) Men put less emphasis on intimacy or emotional closeness and often complain about the infrequency of sexual relations versus a lack of intimacy. The women complain about feeling distant from their partner and the constant threat of abandonment and loneliness (the profession comes first). Men respond to these emotions with their own feelings of being trapped.

The differing needs for intimacy in the medical marriage come, in part, from the clear division of labor (Gabbard & Menninger, 1988). In the traditional medical marriage, the physician husband's role is unequivocally career oriented and the wife concentrates on taking care of the children and home. The physician tends to have his needs met at the workplace. Not only his intellectual needs, but also his needs for companionship, recognition, and intimacy are often met by colleagues and patients. His wife can usually sense the growing distance between her and her husband, but she is busy in the caretaking role and enjoys the advantages of a successful, ambitious spouse. The biggest advantage is economic. Eventually, the division of labor leads to diverging courses of growth and, subsequently, a lack of intimacy, as seen in the following example.

> Dr. J was a successful neurosurgeon at a large, prestigious hospital in the city. He worked 6 days a week, 12 to 14 hours a day for 30 years. Sunday was his only day off, and it was designated "Family Day" and included his wife and four children. He and his wife eventually had only the children and their home in common. She was always active in the children's activities and also

used her spare time to cultivate her interest in photography. The marriage gradually disintegrated and the couple separated. Dr. J entered treatment for chemical dependency and his spouse found a niche in codependent groups and Al-Anon. They made attempts to work on their marriage via marital therapy, individual therapy for both of them, and trials at living together again. They discovered that they had grown in completely different directions as their marriage spanned 3 decades. There had been no intimacy at all during this time. Sex was also infrequent and the wife often described it as "meeting their biological needs."

This couple is still separated after 5 years in recovery. Each has pursued his or her own area of interest, but they continue to procrastinate in ending their marriage legally. This is not unusual. According to research (Vaillant, Sobowale, & McArthur, 1972), physician marriages report more marital discord than other marriages, yet a lower-than-average divorce rate (Rose & Rosow, 1972). This data suggests that medical marriage couples are more tolerant of marital stress and unhappiness when compared with other married couples.

Another reason for the differing needs for intimacy is the different communication styles of the husband and wife. This is related to gender differences and the personality trait of compulsivity in the physician. It appears that the nonphysician wife prefers verbal communication, while physicians tend to use nonverbal actions to express emotion. The emotionally inexpressive physician is rewarded for this behavior in medical school and residency. In the studies of medical marriages by Gabbard and Menninger, physicians' primary complaint is their spouses' lack of sexual interest. This may be a nonverbal response to the lack of intimacy in the marriage. The authors will be comparing some of Menninger and Gabbard's results with their results obtained from recovering medical couples.

INTIMACY IN MEDICAL MARRIAGES WITH CHEMICAL DEPENDENCY

Intimacy and sex problems are prevalent in couples where one or both partners suffer from the disease of chemical dependency. The physician husband may be impotent or rendered physically incapable of sexually performing by an addiction. He also uses most of his energy using his drugs, withdrawing, acquiring the drugs or alcohol, hiding drug use from others, and denying his disease. That leaves very little time and energy for sex and intimacy. Some chemical addictions are coupled with sexual addictions or increased sexuality in the user, but these are acts reduced to biological needs and are void of feelings such as love, tenderness, warmth, and affection.

There is also an emotional component to the lack of intimacy. The physician and spouse are in too much pain to discuss, let alone understand, their feelings. The emotions that are released are usually negative — anger, jealousy, hatred, fear, and shame. It is impossible to be intimate with these feelings acting as a wall between the partners.

A spiritual component to the lack of intimacy is present as well. Both individuals are empty wells. There is no sense of self-awareness, and sexuality is often another manipulation of the need to feel in control of an uncontrollable lifestyle. The addict may abstain from sex to avoid being vulnerable, or out of fear of not being able to perform, or out of anger at the spouse. The addict may demand sex and reduce it to a technical act. The spouse will also abstain from sex for the same reasons. She may carry her caretaking role into the bedroom and have sex when she does not want to, or avoid asking for what she needs. Many codependents lose interest in sex and make up reasons to refrain.

Extramarital affairs are common with chemical dependency. They are often seen as a solution to the loneliness felt in the marriage. Unfortunately, many codependents retreat to another dysfunctional relationship and repeat the same mistakes they made in the first. The problem of intimacy in chemically dependent relationships must begin with healing in each individual before healing as a couple. This healing can come as treatment and a 12-step program for each, focusing on their own needs and pain.

Chemical dependency does not allow intimacy within a couple. A medical marriage already crumbling from the differing needs for intimacy will surely succumb to devastation when this disease is present. The physician and spouse may be less aware of this lack of intimacy because their diverging tracks have left them out of touch with each other. It is often colleagues who will demand a change, even though it is the spouse who will first notice his sickness but choose to put up with it.

RECOVERY AND MEDICAL MARRIAGES

The authors have sought to compare medical marriages and "recovering" medical marriages to determine whether recovery from drugs and alcohol has an impact on the marriage itself. Medical marriages are unique, and alcohol and drug use exaggerates the existing problems in these relationships. What happens when the physician recovers from drug and alcohol dependency? Do their problems lessen? Do these "recovering" couples move to a new level of awareness and definition of their relationship? The authors chose to look at these questions by duplicating some of the questionnaires that Gabbard and Menninger sent to physicians and their spouses and sending them to recovering physicians and their spouses. Only a small part of their study was used, but the results are indeed different.

One hundred questionnaires were sent to physicians and their spouses or significant others. The answers were anonymous and confidential. The questionnaire included a duplication from Gabbard and Menninger's 5-point scale measuring marriage gratification and the top 10 from a list of 15 sources of marital conflict. Each respondent was asked to rate these issues on a scale of 1 to 10, with 1 being the greatest source of conflict and 10 the least. Another list of the top 10 of 12 problems perceived by the marital partner was also sent to be rated on the same scale.

Of the 100 questionnaires, 68 were returned. Only 50 of these were applicable to the study. The physicians were mostly Caucasian men with a mean age of 41 years. The significant others and spouses were mostly Caucasian women divided equally between professionals and homemakers.

The medical specialties of the physicians were varied and included family practice, psychiatry, internal medicine, general surgery, emergency medicine, addictionology, obstetrics-gynecology, anesthesiology, cardiology, oncology, gastroenterology, otolaryngology, and radiology. When the physician was asked the number of hours worked per week, most of them answered 40. Also, the physicians in recovery had 1 to 5 years of sobriety. Most of the physicians in the study by Gabbard and Menninger worked more than 40 hours per week.

The results of Gabbard and Menninger are shown in Table 7-1 for comparison with the authors' results. The results reflect less than half the sample size surveyed by Gabbard and Menninger. Nonetheless, this sample is large enough to make some interesting comparisons.

Gabbard and Menninger gave a possible explanation for the majority of medical marriages being rated as either extremely gratifying or moderately gratifying. They presumed that medical couples have "low expectations or a need to project an image of harmony." They had the added knowledge of knowing which of the couples either sought or considered marital counseling and used this information in their deductions.

The authors' results, in contrast, differed not only with the average physician, but also with the spouse. Most recovering physicians rated their marriage moderately gratifying and mixed. There was also a big discrepancy between the average physician and the recovering physician in that a greater number of recovering doctors rated their marriages "extremely nongratifying" and a smaller number rated them "extremely gratifying." The spouses of recovering physicians had a more varied sample, with the greatest number rating their marriages mixed and none rating their marriages "extremely nongratifying." The recovering sample appeared to be a little more realistic and less concerned with public image, possibly because their images were already tarnished by the stigma of being chemically dependent and so it was easier to be realistic.

Table 7-1.

Rating of Marriage Gratification by Physicians and Their Spouses

	Recovering Physicians (%)		Spouses/Significant Others (%)	
Rating of Marriage Gratification	Gabbard/ Menninger	Authors' Results	Gabbard/ Menninger	Authors' Results
Extremely gratifying	32.8	6.7	28.8	21.0
Moderately gratifying	45.5	40.0	40.8	25.0
Mixed	11.2	40.0	19.2	35.0
Moderately nongratifying	8.2	0	4.8	19.0
Extremely nongratifying	0.8	13.0	4.8	0

It is likely that chemical dependency puts added stress on the marriage and creates more problems for the couple. The spouses react to this disease in various ways. Some are relieved and welcome the recovery process for their spouses and themselves, and others continue to deny its effect on the marriage and choose to ignore it. But if a spouse is unwilling to support her chemically dependent partner she will usually leave the marriage. Therefore, we are assuming that all the spouses of recovering physicians are at least somewhat supportive of the recovery process and committed to the marriage. This may account for the 0% response to "extremely nongratifying."

Table 7-2.

Sources of Conflict Cited by Physicians and Their Spouses

Source of Conflict	Physicians' Ratings (Rank Order)		Spouse/Significant Other's Ratings (Rank Order)	
	Gabbard/ Menninger	Authors' Results	Gabbard/ Menninger	Authors' Results
Lack of time for fun, family, and self	1	9	1	3
Amount of time away from home at work	2	6	8	6
Frequency of sexual relations	3	4	4	4
Finances	4	8	5	5
Money management	5	5	3	7
Tension in the family home	6	2	7	2
Lack of intimacy	7	1	2	1
Lack of shared responsibilities for children and for work around the house	8	7	6	9
Philosophy of child rearing	9	10	9	10
Quality of sexual relations	10	3	10	8

1 = greatest source of conflict; 10 least source of conflict.

Table 7-2 includes part of Gabbard and Menninger's results for comparison with the authors' results. The top 10 of 15 sources of marital conflict in their study were rated on a scale of 1 to 10.

Physicians and spouses ranked sources of conflict fairly similarly; "lack of time for fun, family, and self" was rated 1 by both. The major discrepancies are that physicians rated "amount of time away from home at work" as a greater source of conflict than their spouses, who rated "lack of intimacy" higher than the physician respondents.

Using additional information from their surveys, Gabbard and Menninger (1988) concluded that "lack of time due to the demands of practice seems to be a complaint that serves the function of externalizing the conflicts in the marriage onto factors outside the marriage, but it is not the primary cause of marital dysfunction" (p. 103). They suggest that the problems we talked about earlier—differing needs for intimacy, differing communications styles, and differing perceptions of the problems—are the chief sources of conflict in medical marriages.

In comparison, the recovering couples also tended to rank sources of conflict similarly, more so than nonrecovering couples. The "lack of intimacy" was first and "tension in the family home" was second. If physicians "externalize" conflicts in medical marriages, then we can assume that in recovery the conflicts are no longer externalized but understood for what they really are. All spouses, recovering or not, rated "lack of intimacy" high on their list. Possibly recovering couples communicate more effectively.

The second-ranked conflict for both recovering people was "tension in the home." It seems more likely that these couples have an increased awareness of what is happening in the marriage and experience strife or conflict as a result of this awareness. There may be more verbal communication because of the input of professionals and other chemically dependent families with whom they have contact during the recovery process. The physician in treatment is definitely encouraged to increase his or her personal awareness and feeling state. The fact that spouses of both sets of physicians rated "lack of intimacy" high on their list supports the stereotype that women are more communicative and appear to be more in touch with their feelings. This, of course, is only applicable in traditional medical marriages. The psychological profile of the male physician would also explain the stereotypical roles in the traditional marriage—the verbal, feeling woman and the nonverbal, compulsive man.

The other comparison that deserves comment is the conflict involving frequency of sexual relations. Physicians and spouses of both studies rated this third or fourth in order of importance. Menninger and Gabbard hypothesize that physicians tend to utilize nonverbal actions to express emotion, with sexual activity possibly being one way. Recovering physicians added quality of sexual relations to this top priority, ranking it even higher than frequency (other physicians ranked quality tenth). This supports the premise that recovering physicians expect more out of their relationships, especially when one looks at the "lack of intimacy" rating. The recovery process, which includes specialized treatment for the physicians in this study, emphasizes communication, resocialization, self-examination, and assertiveness (confronting denial of emotional issues). These tools probably overcome some of the earlier described personality traits of the physician, and allow them to be more expressive and in touch with their needs.

The spouse of the recovering physician continues to give a high ranking to lack of time for fun, family, and self. The physician works less and may spend more time at home when recovering, but he nonetheless remains compulsive and unavailable. His compulsion is more self-centered in recovery, involving such focuses as 12-step meetings and nonchemical coping skills (meditation, exercise, etc.).

Gabbard and Menninger found that the primary concern of physicians is that their spouse is not "interested in sex" (Table 7-3). Their spouses primarily complained that their partners did "not talk to them." They concluded that it is probably a communication problem—when the physician wants to have sex the spouse wants to talk. Each partner is left with "unmet emotional needs and the feeling that he or she is misunderstood." This inevitably will lead to marital dissatisfaction.

The comparison of results in this survey illustrated that recovering physicians and both sets of spouses had similar feelings. Again, the recovering couples rated the top two problems the same: first, that the other "doesn't listen to me," and second, that the other "doesn't provide enough emotional support for me." The partners appear to want

Table 7-3.

Importance of Problems Perceived in Marital Partner

Perceived Problem	Physician's Perception of Spouse		Spouse's Perception of Physician	
	Gabbard/ Menninger	Authors' Results	Gabbard/ Menninger	Authors' Results
Is not interested in sexual activity	1	6	9	9
Doesn't empathize with my role and position	2	5	4	3
Doesn't listen to me	3	1	3	1
Expects too much work around the house from me	4	8	8	8
Complains too much	5	4	7	6
Doesn't provide enough emotional support for me	6	2	2	2
Nags me too much about my lack of time at home	7	9	10	10

(continued)

Doesn't talk to me enough	8	3	1	4
Doesn't respect me enough	9	7	5	5
Expects too much from me sexually	10	10	6	7

In rank order
   1 = most serious
   10 = least serious

the same things for themselves, but are not meeting one another's needs.

There are several hypotheses that may explain these results. Recovery is a process of awareness, and a lot of insight becomes available to the participants during this time. It is not always safe to share insights with the partner, mainly because of the relationship's unsafe history during chemical dependency. The individuals may be consumed with their own pain and growth, and cannot listen or provide emotional support for their partners. The spouse of the nonrecovering physician may feel this way due to the lack of time for her and the personality of the physician.

Another interesting point is that the recovering physician moves from the physician's point of view to the spouse's point of view; i.e., their results correlate more with the spouses than the physicians. Maybe they relinquish their "role" for a while and are much more attuned to emotional needs. Sexual activity rates only sixth but is still higher than the rating of ninth by spouses. Recovering doctors are more communicative and rely less on nonverbal actions. They now put more emphasis on talking, as seen with the high rating for "doesn't talk to me."

THE MODEL MEDICAL MARRIAGE

Talbott, through the study of more than 2,500 physicians and their families, developed seven elements that constitute the model medical marriage. We have thus far discussed the unique problems facing the medical marriage, including chemical dependency. Can couples that statistically have the highest rate of dissatisfaction in marriage, improve their relationship, and be role models for happy, healthy marriages? Talbott has witnessed a large number of "redefined and refined medical marriages that can truly be called model marriages." The seven elements of the model medical marriage are categorized here in order of importance.

1. *Partnership Trust.* The healthy marriage must be based on bilateral trust, which is a product of honesty and sharing. In dealing with the healthy model marriage, it quickly becomes apparent that dishonesty is 40% lying, deceiving, and distortion of facts, and 60% hiding or withholding emotions, facts, or events. So often, the illusion that "to let the partner know would hurt them" deceives the relationship and increases the dishonesty. Sharing is critical, for if the partners do not experience each other's anger, resentment, fear, or pain, they cannot truly know each other. To truly trust the partner is to trust their negative and hostile feelings as well as their positive feelings. It must be noted, however, that trust is earned. Therefore, the spouse of a recovering alcoholic needs time to reestablish trust in her partner.

2. *Communication.* This is a special, vulnerable area in medicine because as the physician is taught to practice and then refine his or her role as a professional communicator, personal intimacy is edited out. Too many times, we have heard the complaint that the spouse (or the children) is tired of being dealt with "like a patient." Good professionals swallow feelings, hide their own emotions, and listen intently while they sublimate their personalities within the patient's problems. This is good for the professional, but bad for personal intimacy within the marriage. Communication must be practiced frequently with objective measurements from third parties or peer groups. This is practiced in good model medical marriages.

3. *Priorities and Value Systems within the Marriage.* The delicate balance between work and personal lives must be constantly assessed and monitored. Medicine encourages and even dictates workaholism. This will interfere with and destroy a marriage. The three priorities that frequently tend to be subverted are:

- The personal growth of the physician (physical, emotional, and spiritual)

- The marriage and family

- The job

The pursuit of the medical career tends to reverse these priorities, and unless they are kept in this proper sequence, the ultimate role of the physician cannot be realized, as he must be balanced in his personal as well as his professional life. The profession of medicine constantly wants to emphasize the job, the career, medical advancements, success, and, subsequently, income. Delayed gratification, diminishing periods of time spent with the spouse, the children, on vacations, and in the marriage, helps to justify these false value systems in the medical life. A simple, effective technique is for both the physician and the spouse to post "life's priorities" on the refrigerator door. This helps to keep these priorities straight every day. While acknowledging that the spouse's life may be dominated by children or a job outside the home, and that the physician's life may be dominated by his profession, the couple must maintain the marriage as a paramount priority.

4. *Time Together.* The most frequently asked question is: How do you expect a doctor in medical school, internship, residency, or private practice to have time for his or her spouse, marriage, and children? Having time for nothing but work seems to be the only alternative for many physicians, but there are no victims, only volunteers. Internships, specialties, and types of practice must be chosen with the priority of the medical marriage in mind. More medical schools, house-staff

training programs, and job placement programs are becoming sensitive to the needs of the healthy medical marriage and the importance of providing time for it. A marriage cannot be wholesome if time is not spent together. Togetherness is required for sharing, intimacy, and growing together as a couple. The very system of medicine would dictate that this be delayed or put off. Too often, these delays will destroy a marriage. One renowned chief of medicine at a teaching hospital used to give his house-staff residents a picnic basket and demand that they take their spouses on a picnic lunch once a week. In this way, he was a very effective marital therapist.

5. *Sexual Compatibility.* In the practice of medicine, many physicians deal with the human body daily in examinations and treatment. This practice, in some way, influences (often subconsciously or subliminally) the attitudes and ways that the physician deals with the spouse in their sexual relationship. After hundreds of interviews, it is apparent that physicians do not freely and openly discuss sexual subjects with their spouses. The manner, intensity, and duration of sexual foreplay was found to be absent in discussions in a large number of medical marriages. There was an integration in the mind of the physician between the spouse and the patient. The "taking for granted" and "I assume" attitudes, which so many spouses volunteered to the authors and therapists, were major problems in the relationship. On the other hand, in the model medical marriage, open discussion about sex, sexual practices, and ongoing discussions about sexual pleasures were a very important component of the healthy union. Our culture gives mixed messages about sexual practices, but open communication about sexual issues will destroy fallacies and misunderstandings. When open discussions were not present in a medical marriage, serious sexual problems often resulted.

6. *Interest in Each Other's Friends and Activities.* One of the most common complaints from spouses is that their physician partner cannot talk about anything except medicine, and his or her friends can only discuss the practice, the patients, or the hospital. Additionally, the activities and friends of the spouse seem trivial and insignificant compared with the physician's daily life-and-death struggles. This not only demeans the spouse, but it hurts the medical marriage. Additionally, this imbalance, in which medicine dominates the physician's life, hurts his or her own spiritual and emotional growth and physical life outside the profession. Reading and understanding nonmedical books is as important as reading the latest medical texts and journals. Analysis of data on the model medical marriage demonstrates that physicians showing greater interest and involvement in their spouse's activities, friends, and projects have stronger marriages. The spouse may respond by being involved in the medical auxiliary or the practice. The couple is then better able to assume an ideal reciprocal relationship. Increasingly, enlightened chiefs of services at teaching hospitals are requesting that the spouses of newlywed members of their house staff spend 24 hours at the hospital, sleeping there and accompanying their husbands or wives for a full day on the job, so they might better understand all aspects of the medical life. This is being done in a number of the specialties. Again, it reverts to the basic principles of communication, sharing, and trust.

7. *Reassessment and Reevaluation of the Marriage Components.* A physician's life and relationships are not static. They change dramatically and profoundly with the changes in his or her professional career. Commitments, promises, and interests may be valid in the beginning, but subject to change when career, job placement, and aging occur. It is important, therefore, to constantly recheck and reassess the components that determine a healthy model medical marriage. This cannot be done subjectively; it requires

third-party objectivity. Workshops and peer groups dealing with the medical marriage are proving very effective. Counselors and marriage therapists are available and effective when individual therapy is indicated. Review of data in the ideal model medical marriages indicates that a large number of these couples are involved in periodic workshops or peer-group reviews of their relationships.

PHYSICIAN-PHYSICIAN MARRIAGES

When both partners in the medical marriage are physicians, certain issues come to the forefront and are exaggerated with chemical dependency. We mention this only to acknowledge the uniqueness of physician-physician marriages. (We will not be addressing this topic in this book.) For example, parenting and professional roles have to be carefully delineated. It is recommended that these issues be examined in the treatment process for both the patient and family member.

SUMMARY

Physicians and their spouses in traditional medical marriages (with the husband the physician) face unique problems related to the personality profile of the physician and the demands of practice, in addition to the problems common in all marriages. The problems are exaggerated with chemical dependency and further reduce satisfaction and gratification in medical marriages. Denial and the willingness to stay in the marriage despite a high level of dissatisfaction is common. The reasons for staying may be financial or involve low self-esteem of the spouse or the need to maintain a high standing in the community. The reasons for dissatisfaction are typically problems in communication and differing needs for intimacy. The main difference between medical marriages with and without recovery from chemical dependency are how these problems are perceived.

It appears that medical couples not in recovery generally tend to externalize the conflicts in their marriage, while couples with one or more years of recovery from chemical dependency correctly identify the real sources of conflict, i.e., lack of communication and intimacy in their marriage. One can hypothesize from these findings that all medical marriages are similar and suffer from a lack of communication and intimacy. However, the process of recovery in chemical dependency enhances the ability of the partners to recognize the problems and to look at the marriage more honestly.

According to research, however, this honesty does not appear to increase satisfaction in the marriage. The process of recovery is based on self-examination and self-honesty and does not focus on the couple, though there are certainly elements that enable the couple to decrease dissatisfaction and work toward the goal of a model medical marriage. These seven elements include trust, communication, priorities, time together, sexuality, outside interests, and time to reevaluate the marriage on a regular basis.

8

Special Issues
for Women Physicians

I never wanted to be a drug addict.
All I ever wanted to be was a doctor.
(Morrison, 1989)

Women constituted 37% of students at American medical schools in 1988 (Bickel), yet only 9% of the professors on medical school faculties were women in 1990 (Tesch, Wood, Helwig, & Butler-Nattinger, 1995). This lack of female role models and mentors in medicine gives women a greater sense of isolation than men. This isolation also results from hostility from the majority (men) and perceived role deviance. Women are still expected to perform their domestic roles of homemaker and mother, even when they choose a demanding profession such as medicine. They often experience an internal struggle because of the dichotomy between their femininity and the traditionally male qualities needed to succeed in this career (AMA, 1986). The isolation felt by women physicians may contribute to the high suicide rate among this minority. Female physicians are four times more likely to commit suicide than women in the general population older than age 25 years (Blachly, Disher, & Roduner, 1968). This is a depressing statistic, but it presents an even more desperate situation when the disease of chemical dependency is introduced.

WOMEN PHYSICIANS AND CHEMICAL DEPENDENCY

Chemically dependent women generally feel more isolated and are more secretive than men. They complain more about insomnia and exhibit feelings of hopelessness, insecurity, mistrust, and self-hatred. They are more prone to depression and have a higher incidence of unstable marriages and divorces than chemically dependent men (Corrigan, 1980). Extramarital affairs are more common in chemically dependent women. There is also a greater incidence of alcoholism in their families of origin (Marsh, Colten, & Tucker, 1982).

When the chemically dependent woman is a physician, the problem list grows to include conflicts over early life experiences and relationships and thwarted expectations in the field of medicine (Martin & Talbott, 1986). They frequently have encountered major traumatic events in their lives prior to treatment for chemical dependency. The death of a significant other and acts of violence directed toward either themselves or their children are among the traumas most frequently cited (Martin & Talbott, 1987). Relapse is often associated with anniversary dates of traumatic events.

As desperate as their lives become, addicted female physicians usually find obstacles to treatment. Interventions for chemically dependent female physicians are much more difficult to accomplish than for male physicians. The stigma associated with alcoholism and drug addiction persists for women. Evidence of this is the fact that most jokes about alcoholics are about men. There is a greater tendency to label alcohol and drug problems in women doctors as a secondary condition to a primary psychoneurosis, whereas the alcohol and drug addiction is considered a primary diagnosis in men (Vincent, 1976). Women doctors are also less likely than men to reach chemical dependency treatment through intervention or peer confrontation; they are stigmatized more than men, so a medical colleague might prefer to diagnose a woman as depressed rather than alcoholic (Bissell & Skorina, 1987). Martin and Talbott (1987) noted that many female physicians have had numerous psychiatric admissions prior to treatment for chemical dependency.

CHALLENGES WOMEN FACE

The special issues experienced by alcohol- and drug-addicted women physicians are painfully expressed in this passage:

> Although I had perfected my exterior persona, I still experienced excruciating inner pain, but I never revealed it to anyone. Rarely a day went by when I didn't experience terror, loneliness, paranoia, and confusion, and I remained preoccupied with death. I just got loaded continuously to cover it all up. (Morrison, 1989)

Dr. Morrison admits feeling "terror." Martin and Talbott (1987) found that the most frequently expressed issues for these women in treatment is "dealing with fear and learning to trust." The breakdown of relationships begins early for most of these women. Fifty-three percent were adult children of alcoholics (Martin & Talbott, 1986), and growing up in a dysfunctional family meant that their relationships were earmarked by boundary distortions and enmeshment. As children they quickly learned that survival means never "rocking the boat." The only thing they learned to trust were secrets, especially as they relate to chemical dependency. They experienced fear of physical and/or emotional harm and retained this fear and lack of trust through adulthood.

CREATING AN ILLUSION

There is a split between who these physicians really are and how they portray themselves to others. They are women in a male dominated field, although that is rapidly changing. "Chemically dependent women often report adapting the traditional female role in the extreme, believing that they do not measure up and that by consciously working and being 'super feminine' they will thereby enhance their poor self-concept and improve dysfunctional relationships" (Martin & Talbott, 1987). Thus, they experience both internal and external conflict. The true self is again denied to please and control the environment around them.

Dr. Morrison also describes feeling "loneliness" and "excruciating inner pain" while using drugs and alcohol. This does not go away in treatment but tends to resurface with self-disclosure. These feelings are often accompanied by a sense of rage at having been used and rejected by significant others in childhood (Martin & Talbott, 1987). The women also express rage at being considered by society as especially deviant in their chemical dependence and in their attempts to achieve and be accepted in a male dominated profession (Martin & Talbott, 1987).

TREATMENT ISSUES

Treatment issues for women have traditionally centered on building trust and dealing with anger, but they also focus on establishing identity and resolving confusion and conflict over sex roles. The "paranoia and confusion" that Dr. Morrison experienced may have been related to the side effects or toxicity of the chemicals she used. But these feelings continue in treatment because of the need to develop clear boundaries and an identity in her role as a woman physician.

Men in recovery talk about needing to dispose of their "oversized egos" and look outside themselves to achieve a proper focus for their lives. Most women describe a fragmented ego and having to look to others in the past for a definition of themselves. They seem to be on a continuous search for sexual and professional validation and often see themselves as victims in relationships and the field of medicine. An important task in recovery for these women is the development of a spiritual program and a sisterhood with other recovering women.

Even in programs that specialize in the treatment of physicians, women are a minority. It is more important that they are able to identify with their gender rather than their occupation. They also need a higher power in their lives that is not a significant other, so they can begin to let go of the burden of control and learn to trust themselves and others. This has proven to be difficult for many women physicians. Expressing overwhelming feelings of unworthiness and shame, they often return to environments devoid of adequate emotional and financial support. Anger and lack of trust also become emotional obstacles for women physicians in treatment. There is a correlation between prolonged residential treatment for physicians and good treatment outcome, but for women the good outcome may come at a higher price (Bissell & Skorina, 1987). Many lose their spouses, children, friends, and jobs, finding their only support in the treatment or the 12-step community. Also, many women continue to report "extreme loneliness" after treatment (Martin & Talbott, 1986).

A sizable number of chemically dependent women physicians do maintain sobriety and make peace with their limited relationships, utilizing available resources. They form networks that consist of people with whom they can identify and from whom they can accept help, regardless of sex and/ or occupation. They remain active in 12-step programs and commit themselves to sober living and spiritual growth. Finally, they become a resource for others, as Dr. Morrison has.

The impaired physicians movement is encouraging, but it must be improved to better meet the needs of women physicians. There must be a greater representation of women on impaired physician committees, and more education and awareness by the medical profession to avoid misdiagnosing chemical dependency as depression (Bissell & Skorina, 1987).

The earlier in one's career the intervention takes place, the better. Each year more women enter medical schools and more women physicians will suffer from chemical dependency. We must recognize their special issues and continue to support and advocate their roles in medicine. Finally, we must be aware of the growing need for women physician mentors in both medicine and the recovering medical community.

The three case studies that follow illustrate some of the chemical dependency issues discussed in this chapter.

Case 1

A 36-year-old female physician in her final year of surgical residency had a family history of alcoholism. Her father was a violent alcoholic and abandoned the family while she was in elementary school. She began to drink alcohol at the age of 15 and gradually experimented with other drugs, including cocaine. She had a few close relationships that she described as dysfunctional and had lived alone for the past 5 years. She entered treatment for chemical dependency when she was found diverting drugs at her hospital. She admitted being very depressed, with thoughts of suicide. Her initial behavior in treatment indicated a need to please others and be well liked by the other patients. Within a few weeks, she relapsed on alcohol and was transferred to another treatment center. At this new facility, she finally surrendered to the diagnosis of chemical dependency, admitting her problem. Her major issues in treatment were shame, poor self-esteem, and abandonment. She successfully completed treatment and has remained an active member of AA and Caduceus aftercare groups. She returned feeling pleased about this decision. She lives with another recovering alcoholic woman and is engaged to a physician who is not chemically dependent.

Case 2

A 38-year-old female physician was not practicing medicine as a result of the consequences of her addiction to drugs and alcohol. She was the oldest child in a family of three with no history of alcoholism. She was sexually abused by her cousins from age 4 to 16 and developed an inherent distrust of men, continuing to have problems with relationships throughout her life. She described herself as an overachiever and a perfectionist with low self-esteem. She only felt good about herself when she was able to achieve educational goals, which prompted her to go to medical school.

Her first experience with alcohol was in college, when she drank until she passed out. She stopped using alcohol in medical school, but during her residency in emergency medicine she began using amphetamines to stay awake. She started to drink and use drugs heavily during the next several years of her residency. She was charged with driving under the influence, began to purchase street drugs (particularly cocaine), and was writing prescriptions for herself and friends. She also lived with a physically abusive man during this time. Two years later, a pharmacist turned her in for inappropriate prescription writing to the authorities and she lost her DEA number. She moved to another city and continued to practice emergency medicine without her DEA number. It was there that one of the nurses introduced her to intravenous cocaine. It gave her a feeling of control and euphoria. She began to isolate herself more and more and used cocaine at work. She suffered many broken bones and black eyes at the hands of her abusive boyfriend. She was finally fired by the director of the emergency department. She got a job in a factory earning only minimum wage and resorted to stealing to support her drug habit. She was charged with two felonies: possession of cocaine and drug paraphernalia. The state medical board received her name, contacted her, and recommended treatment at two centers that specialize in treating physicians. After becoming suicidal, she finally called one of the treatment programs for help.

She stayed in treatment for 8 months; at first she was very resistant, but later became an active member of the recovering community. Six months later the board gave her permission to practice medicine again. This was difficult for her because she had a lot of shame and did not feel totally accepted as both a female physician and a recovering drug addict. She continues to successfully practice medicine and is an active member of AA.

Case 3

A 42-year-old anesthesiologist had a family history of alcoholism (mother), and her father committed suicide when she was a young child. She stated she is close to her mother and boyfriend but has no other friends. She had a strict religious upbringing and was never encouraged to develop hobbies or social skills as a child. The patient first used alcohol at age 17, but heavy drug use did not begin until medical school and residency. This was a woman who was always at the top of her class, a high achiever. She became aware that she had a drinking problem when she found herself getting drunk every night and always alone. She also realized that she most wanted to use drugs when feelings of guilt and anger arose in her. Her drug use extended to stimulants, morphine, hydrocodone, cocaine, and finally fentanyl. She was recommended for treatment after an intervention by the head of anesthesia and other operating room staff. In treatment, the patient was emotionally guarded, defensive, and angry. As time went on, she began to make meaningful relationships in treatment and develop a program in AA. She also had difficulty identifying herself as anything other than a doctor. The patient worked on this and other issues in treatment and eventually was discharged. She chose to leave the field of anesthesia and began a residency in psychiatry. Today she is still sober and successfully practicing psychiatry.

9

The Family and Codependency

All families fall somewhere on a continuum from "very nurturing" to "very troubled." The atmosphere in a troubled family is easy to sense (Satir, 1988). Members of troubled families may experience feelings of discomfort, secrecy, and superficiality, or feel as if they are "walking on eggshells," which is a typical description from family members in alcoholic homes. These descriptions cover only a small part of what is really going on (Satir, 1988). Family members may suspect more than what they see and hear, but are fearful or unsure about finding out just how troubled their family is. In the alcoholic home, family members are often afraid to "rock the boat" and set their family on a dangerous course; but in order to become nurturing, the family must recognize that it is troubled and take the risk to change (see Table 9-1).

Denial is the defense mechanism most often employed by family members to cope with dysfunction and negative feelings. The members also defend against the pathology by role playing. These roles include (Wegscheider-Cruse, 1990):

Table 9-1.

Characteristics of an Alcoholic Home

Centricity of alcoholism/addiction and associated behaviors
Denial and shame
Inconsistency, insecurity, and fear
Anger and hate
Guilt and blame
Parent—child role reversals
Lack of role models for dealing with stress
Lack of joy and fun
Helplessness and loss of control

1. *The Enabler.* This is usually a spouse who, in order to feel needed and keep the peace, enables a partner to continue drinking or using drugs and assume that he is meeting the expectations of a supportive partner. Other family members or main significant others can also take on the role of enabler.

2. *The Hero.* Often the eldest child, this person struggles to be perfect so that the family will look good to others.

3. *The Scapegoat.* This may be a child whose antisocial behavior becomes the focal point and distracts attention away from the alcoholic.

4. *The Lost Child.* This child may deny the problem by "fading into the woodwork" (i.e., watching excessive television, spending excessive time on computer work, video games, etc.) and isolating in order to decrease or avoid tension in the family.

5. *The Mascot.* This family member covers up the pain by being charming and humorous.

Family rules, spoken or unspoken, perpetuate the troubled family system. These rules discourage communication and intimacy, and since they do not foster growth, the relationships they affect become rigid, mistrustful, and dysfunctional. Many such rules, as listed in Table 9-2, can be recognized by their opening words "Do not" (Subby, 1990).

In general, family members who grow up with these rulesstruggle with identity problems or codependency as adults.

Table 9-2.

Rules That Perpetuate the Troubled Family System

'Do not talk about problems or feelings
`Do not feel
"Do not trust
"Do not touch
Do not make mistakes
Do not be selfish
Do not rock the boat
Do not have fun
Do not talk about sex
Do not be yourself
°One of the four main rules.

MEDICAL FAMILIES

Many medical families, while not dealing with chemical dependency, may nevertheless identify with the rules, roles, and characteristics that are found in chemically dependent families. In general, a physician's personality is earmarked by compulsivity, which tends to decrease intimacy and increase workaholism and other compulsive behaviors. Spouses and children frequently center their lives on the physician and learn to have their needs met outside the family system. When the physician is chemically dependent, the same rules and roles become exaggerated. Denial and the conspiracy of silence allow the physician to progress in the disease. Family members are also deterred from seeking outside help due to other factors, such as loss of income, fear of malpractice, loss of status, and the misguided view that health professionals can heal themselves.

As discussed in Chapter 7, the spouse and physician have a high rate of dissatisfaction in their marriage due to lack of communication and differing needs for intimacy (the physician's need is usually less). The spouse adapts to a partner who does not communicate, is nonverbal, works too much, and uses sex, primarily, to meet intimacy needs at home. When the physician becomes chemically dependent, the spouse feels even more isolated. She may try to confront the chemically dependent physician but she may be met with anger, denial, or increased time away from home. The spouse sees only two options: leave the alcoholic or keep the peace. This behavior is part of a three-stage illness the spouse experiences while the physician is abusing drugs and alcohol. Most spouses choose to keep the peace and become increasingly responsible and enabling. They become the "silent, solicitous caretaker." This is the first stage.

Stage 2 is the "disease of codependency." The spouse tries to please all the people in her life all the time, feels responsible for everyone's thoughts and feelings, has no sense of her own identity, has difficulty expressing feelings or maintaining intimate relationships, and becomes inflexible. During this stage, physical symptoms and illness may develop or progress, together with an emotional and spiritual bankruptcy. The spouse's tragedy is that she simply lacks knowledge and awareness of chemical dependency and believes that the alcoholic could stop with a little willpower. She feels angry and ashamed, but helpless because she does not feel safe talking about the problem.

Stage 3 for the "spousoholic" is grief. Psychiatrist Elizabeth Kibler-Ross (1969) lists five stages of grief: denial, anger, bargaining, depression, and acceptance. People grieve for losses, whatever they may be. The spouse of an alcoholic grieves the loss of healthy and nurturing relationship and family. She grieves the loss of her physician husband who is chemically dependent.

STAGES OF GRIEF

When an alcoholic health professional enters treatment, the spouse or significant other is usually in some stage of grief.

The first stage of grief is denial. The spouse in denial will frequently refuse to be involved in a family program at a treatment center or support group. She may say that it's not her problem, or say, "If we can just get rid of this weakness, we'll be all right." If the spouse can be persuaded to attend Al-Anon or other support groups, she may just sit silently and "feel sorry" for the other members. Unfortunately, this behavior helps keep the family on the "troubled" end of the family continuum. Denial can be overcome through awareness, education, role models, and an opportunity to talk and listen to others in her situation. Remember, this is a defense mechanism employed by the spouse for protection. She must feel safe in order to give it up.

It is always gratifying to hear a spouse come to a support group and express anger — the second stage of grief. This implies that the spouse is aware of a problem and feels the ramifications. Many angry group members have difficulty maintaining a genuine relationship with the alcoholic because of a history of abuse, hurt, and shame. As insurmountable as this may seem, the spouse gradually begins to feel free of this anger as she is able to express her feelings to "safe" people. Safe people are those who understand and empathize with people suffering from the diseases of chemical dependency and codependency, and who agree to confidentiality. More than likely, this will not be the addicted spouse. Impaired partners often experience too much pain early in recovery to support their spouses. The empathy in support groups for significant others of impaired health professionals is twofold: all are in a relationship with a physician or other highly accountable health professional and all are experiencing the disease of chemical dependency.

The third stage of grief is bargaining. This is exemplified by an impaired physician's spouse who came to a support group and stated that she would continue to come to these groups only if her alcoholic husband would get better. It is no cause for disappointment when a new member joins the group as a bargaining tool. Eventually, through the group process, the spouse identifies with other group members and begins to enthusiastically attend the group for her issues. Other bargains can be between the spouse and God, the physician, children, etc.

Depression is the fourth stage of grief. The depression a spouse feels may or may not need psychiatric intervention. Regardless of the severity of the feelings, depression is a painful state. Depression in spouses can manifest itself in a number of ways, including lack of motivation, depressed affect, physical problems, and loss of interest in appearance, activities, or family life. Telephone contact and support persons can assist the depressed spouse in expressing feelings and finding others who can empathize with her. Gradually the depression lifts and may be replaced by anger or relief.

The final stage of grief is acceptance. Eventually, there is acceptance that the diseases of codependency and chemical dependency are part of their lives. For instance, a spouse may know she has accepted that she has an alcoholic spouse when she no longer needs to deny the diagnosis to others. She accepts that he is an addict and an alcoholic, and it is no longer an uncomfortable fact.

The stages of grief do not always occur in sequence and a spouse may experience one stage several times. One spouse of an impaired nurse often talks about "triggers" that bring back waves of depression, guilt, and anger even years into recovery. The feelings are short lived but nonetheless painful and uncomfortable.

Communication is the key to both medical marriages and the recovery process. Because most medical couples have no history of sustained, open, honest communication, it is difficult to institute such communication during recovery. Recovery begins with communication outside the family system. Al-Anon is an exceptional source of support and in- formation for the spouse and family. But because medical families are part of the conspiracy of silence, feeling the need to protect the impaired physician or health care worker from malpractice suits or the loss of medical license, income, or status, most spouses of addicted health professionals are too fearful to attend Al-Anon. Both the Illinois and the Georgia programs discussed in Chapter 2 are unique in that they provide groups for significant others of health professionals. These are not 12-step groups, but supportive-learning groups led by qualified therapists. They are confidential and allow significant others to express forbidden thoughts, feelings, and experiences, without fearing reprisal. This is often the first time spouses talk about the chemical dependency in their families. It is common for these significant others to attend Al-Anon only after a positive experience in these support groups.

Some state medical societies, such as those in Florida, Oklahoma, and Indiana, have developed medical family programs that include education, support networks, structured facilitated groups, referral to appropriate programs and resources, and confidentiality.

Individual and marital—family therapy are often recommended. The best chance of success comes with a therapist who has experience in treating chemical dependency in families. The process of self-examination and/or treatment is best accomplished "one day at a time." Recovery is a lifetime process and not an event. It is estimated that the alcoholic and his or her spouse may devote 1 to 2 years to their own recovery before working on other relationships in the marriage and family. Although this is an individual preference and need, it is important to note that unless the self is healed, other relationships will remain wounded.

HELP FOR THE CHILDREN

Help for children in chemically dependent families is always recommended following solid recovery programs for both parents. It has been noted that children will begin to show signs of increased health and well-being even without specific intervention, as they begin to feel and model the serenity being experienced by their recovering parents. However, simple and honest communication is very important. Children in recovery must hear and believe four key messages:

1. You are not alone.

2. It's not your fault.

3. Chemically dependent people can and do recover.

4. You need to help yourself.

To help the children, one must help them understand chemical dependency. Explain the disease in simple terms and allow them the opportunity to attend community or treatment center education seminars, if appropriate.

Children must be helped to feel better about themselves. Feelings of self-esteem can only flourish in an atmosphere in which individual differences are appreciated, love is shown openly, mistakes are used for learning, communication is open, rules are flexible, responsibility is modeled, and honesty is practiced, i.e., the kind of atmosphere found in a nurturing family (Satir, 1988). Parents can pass feelings of value and appreciation on to their children not only in what they say but how they say it.

Children need help to evaluate constructive coping options. They need to learn to express feelings, to not let drinking and drug use interfere with things that are important to them, and to stay out of parental arguments. Finally, children need to learn trust through consistency and time. There are also 12-step programs for children and adolescents (e.g., Ala-Teen) that offer peer support and recovery. Rush has a specific program for children. It is a $2^1/2$ day treatment which offers education and allows children to express their thoughts and feelings in a safe and therapeutic environment. The children are very receptive.

As the patient, spouse, and children consistently focus on self, learn to communicate openly and honestly, and increase flexibility of family rules, the family system moves up the continuum toward nurturing. The air of secrecy and discomfort begins to dissipate.

Dysfunctional family roles are relinquished when members are appreciated and esteemed for their individual differences. It is a long, arduous road, but well worth the effort. After several months in recovery, many spouses have stated that they were grateful to be married to someone recovering from chemical dependency, saying that without the disease, they would never have had the opportunity for self-discovery and a healthy family life.

CODEPENDENCY

It is essential to discuss codependency in a book about chemical dependency. It has become a popular term over the past decades as the result of overidentification, quick fixes, and an abundance of self-help books on the subject. Many psychiatrists and other mental health professionals are skeptical and often critical of the term due to its cultlike nature. We have opened as well as closed codependency treatment programs because of the backlash from this movement. However, people who have grown up with an addict or alcoholic or live as an adult with this disease share some common characteristics. They also can recover with the help of 12-step programs and qualified psychotherapists. It is our experience that codependency must not be overemphasized or underemphasized, but confronted as part of the family disease of addiction.

Codependency has been described as a disease, a personality disorder, and an illness. Many authors have developed theoretical frameworks of codependence, but these have only added to the confusion and skepticism of people in the mental health professions or those searching for personal growth. Wegscheider-Cruse (1990) illustrates the difficulty in defining codependency using the parable of the blind men and the elephant. In this story, each of the blind men was asked to feel and describe an elephant standing directly in front of him. Each gave an accurate yet totally different description, but none actually suggested it was an elephant.

Despite the existence of conflicting theories, the main contributors in the field of codependency have agreed on a definition: codependency is a pattern of painful dependency on compulsive behaviors and approval from others in an attempt to find safety, self-worth, and identity (Schaef, 1986); recovery is possible, they add.

Family members affected by the disease of chemical dependency are often described as codependent. Their lives are focused outside themselves in an effort to deny and survive the chaos of addiction. The signs and symptoms of codependency are listed in Table 9-3. When family members break through the denial of their dependency on people, places, or things, the process of healing can begin.

Table 9-3.

Signs and Symptoms of Codependency

Denial
Lack of self-worth
Caretaking to the exclusion of one's own needs
Inability to identify personal feelings and needs
Difficulty communicating
People-pleasing or need for others' approval
Feeling responsible for others' behavior
Telling a lie when the truth would be easier
Use of compulsive behaviors to avoid focusing on self (e.g., excessive shopping, workaholism, excessive exercise)
Need to feel in control
Difficulty setting limits or boundaries
Anxiety
Depression
Perfectionism

Health professionals, especially those affected or afflicted with the disease of chemical dependency, may also exhibit signs and symptoms of codependency. The health professions reward some of the codependent behaviors that allow untreated professionals to continue denying the adverse effects of codependency on their lives. Nurses and physicians are beginning to recognize this dysfunction in themselves. The case studies that follow will more fully characterize codependent behavior.

Case 1

A nurse in an intensive care unit works overtime despite her physiological need for sleep. She is caring for two postoperative cardiac patients, both of whom need continuous observation, physical care, and specialized monitoring. She is aware that she has skipped a meal and needs a bathroom break, but is afraid to leave her patients. She fears that another nurse will not be prepared for a potential crisis or may not be able to maintain the current status of her patients. Once in a while she thinks about her personal life, but quickly puts these thoughts aside because of the important task at hand. She is far too busy to engage in idle talk with other staff members. She feels anger when she overhears them laughing while at the nurse's station. She finishes the second shift in silence and rushes to ensure that her patients and their bedsides are in order before reporting to the next shift. While driving home, she desperately tries to think of something she may have forgotten to do or report.

This nurse represents more the rule than the exception, especially in critical care nursing. She exhibits the four main behaviors common to all codependent health professionals.

The first behavior is caretaking. She is caring for the needs of others to the exclusion of her own. She neglects her needs to eat, sleep, and urinate. She also neglects her need to have a personal life outside of her profession. She feels that she alone is responsible for these patients' lives. Part of the reward for the nurse is a sense of control. Her personal life may seem so out of control that she overcompensates at work to regain some self-esteem. She also refuses to trust a colleague enough to take a break; then she feels like a martyr. Codependents believe they are suffering for a good cause and that they are admired for suffering.

Snow and Willard (1989) found that 93% of nurses responding to their survey are dealing with self-esteem issues. They are able to obtain a strong sense of value when caring for others, so they are generally overcommitted and overworked. The low self-esteem felt by this large percentage of nurses can lead to perfectionism, which is the second behavior manifested by codependent health professionals.

Perfectionism, often exhibited by being rigid, judgmental and controlling, is frequently encouraged in health care delivery systems. Physicians and nurses are urged to keep up with paperwork, "fix" patients, and support and appease family members. The continuous threats of malpractice and rigid time schedules also can promote perfectionism.

Case 2

Dr. Z practices surgery at a teaching hospital in a large city. Her many responsibilities include patient care, teaching, keeping up to date with current medical research and technology, and office duties. She struggles to do all of these perfectly, perpetuating the illusion that she is in total control. She is aware that nurses and ancillary staff have labeled her as arrogant, but fears that if she lets her guard down she will lose control. Her self-esteem needs are met by being needed and getting the job done. Her relationships have historically been dysfunctional and painful, so she isolates herself from colleagues and family. Eventually, drugs and alcohol become her escape from the loneliness and pain.

The sad reality is that Dr. Z denies there is anything wrong in her life. The third codependent behavior, denial, is one of the most prevalent defense mechanisms employed by codependents and addicts. Dr. Z avoids the difficulties and pain in her personal life by keeping busy in her professional life. Denial of feelings leads to a progressive inability to realize any feelings at all. Codependents become so preoccupied in fulfilling the expectations of others that they lose their own identity. The compulsive personality of physicians also contributes to these behaviors.

The fourth behavior common to codependent health professionals is poor communication. All of these behaviors and characteristics are related through poor communication. For someone who is focused outside of self (external referenting), is rigid and a perfectionist, and denies feelings, honest communication will be difficult. Codependents tend to communicate in ways that are judgmental, shameful, and dishonest. One sign of codependency is telling a lie when telling the truth would be easier. This next case illustrates this symptom.

Case 3

A nurse on a busy medical surgical unit had worked 7 consecutive days. He had 1 day off and was then scheduled to work another 4 days. He was physically exhausted, but felt guilty about calling the unit to request more time off. Instead, he called the nursing registry and said he was ill with the flu and a temperature of 103° (F). It would have been just as easy to state the truth, that he was physically exhausted, but he did not feel this was reason enough to warrant leaving the unit short-staffed. He lied because of his shame and later felt guilty about his dishonesty.

Codependency in health professionals, especially nurses, is often rewarded by the profession. Caretaking, perfectionism, denial, and even poor communication are behaviors that help focus on patient care and ignore the needs of the caregiver. Initially, everyone is happy. The patient is given optimal treatment and the nurse or physician is highly satisfied with his or her work. As time goes on, however, feelings of anger, shame, and resentment creep into the professional demeanor of the caregiver. These feelings are directed toward themselves, authority figures, institutions, and family members. The result is burnout. Traditionally, nurses who experience burnout may look for another job, perhaps in another profession, whereas physicians begin to isolate from family and focus all their energy onto their careers.

There is another potential consequence of codependency and burnout. Health care professionals often turn to drugs and alcohol to ease the pain. If they have the predisposition for the disease of chemical dependency, there is a good chance they will cross the boundary into addiction. Given the availability of powerful narcotics, some caregivers will experiment with mood-altering chemicals. In a short period of time, the health care professional is jeopardizing family, career, and patient care to acquire his or her drug of choice.

Addiction is a life-threatening disease and therefore immediate treatment for chemical dependency is critical. Once the health care professional has successfully completed treatment and is recovering, the issue of codependency is often overlooked. If codependent behaviors are not addressed and healthy behaviors are not pursued, the recovering caregiver may relapse or use another addictive process to escape the pain. The pain is often the product of codependent behavior—feelings of shame, anger, and low self-esteem. The mirror-image placement phase in the Talbott and Rush programs require the addict to identify and confront these behaviors. This is a beginning, but many addicts and alcoholics require further intervention after treatment.

Wegscheider-Cruse (1990) believes that "if you scratch the paint off a substance abuser . . . you find a 'behavioral' abuser."

She adds that most alcoholics have "coexisting dependencies." Behaviors that become compulsive and dysfunctional include:

- Workaholism
- Compulsive eating
- Compulsive caretaking and controlling others
- Sexual acting out
- Spending and gambling
- Excessive exercise
- "Guru chasing" (chasing the newest method of self-help at any cost)

Again, two of these behaviors, workaholism and caretaking, are rewarded in the health professions. The others are often regarded as the lesser of two evils (not as bad as the disease of chemical dependency). The recovering alcoholic-addict continues to deny or numb uncomfortable thoughts and feelings through the pursuit of these behavioral "medicators" (Wegscheider-Cruse, 1990). This leads to isolation, shame, low self-esteem, and an inability to maintain loving relationships. The result is often medical problems, relationship problems, and relapse. Relapse in the health professional can be so devastating that suicide is often considered a solution. Therefore, we must consider the health professional untreated unless recovery includes confronting issues in codependency.

RECOVERY FROM CODEPENDENCY

The codependent individual's ability to identify compulsive or dysfunctional behaviors and traits is key to recovery. The mirror-image phase in chemical dependency treatment, family programs and groups, and 12-step meetings are opportunities to achieve this. But the individual must also be willing to surrender or take the first step—to admit powerlessness over other people and behaviors (Table 9-4). This is a gradual process. There are often feelings of anger, pain, resentment, and grief during this time, which may warrant intervention by an experienced counselor or group leader.

Table 9-4.

The Codependent's Part in the Recovery Process

Attending 12-step meetings or other appropriate support groups
Applying the steps and other recovery concepts to their lives
Working with a therapist, if appropriate
Attending seminars and workshops
Maintaining an attitude of honesty, openness, and willingness to try
Struggling through the frustration, awkwardness, and discomfort of change
Connecting with other recovering people
Reading meditation books and other helpful literature
Continuing to surrender

From Beattie, 1989.

Codependency or behavioral treatment offers a safe environment and small group process to express feelings and confront core issues. Treatment for codependency is offered via actual treatment programs or outpatient psychotherapy. It is important that the treatment team and therapists understand the disease of chemical dependency and its effect on the entire family, that the codependent be able to identify with others who feel and behave as they do, and that he or she attend 12-step groups on a regular basis.

Health care professionals need not abandon the qualities that make them successful. It is a matter of distinguishing when a behavior or trait is used to avoid feelings and isolate oneself from relationships. It is imperative that these behaviors and traits be identified and attempts made to understand and change them. Again, this is a process and not an event. Recovering individuals must be gentle with themselves throughout recovery and allow others to support and nurture them along the way.

It is often helpful for the family members to have guidelines regarding their own recovery. Listed in Table 9-5 are phases of recovery that the main significant other usually experiences following the patient's admission to a chemical dependency treatment program. It has been helpful to significant others to understand their fears, needs, and development during the treatment of a loved one.

Table 9-5.

DRAFT and DRAG Phases of Recovery for Significant Others in Chemical Dependency'

After Admission to Treatment Program (DRAFT)		
D	Despair	The significant others initially feel "despair" when they give up their loved one to a treatment program. Many are tearful and feel overwhelming loneliness and fear of the future.
R	Relief	Several days to weeks after the chemically dependent loved one has been in treatment, there is a welcome feeling of relief. They no longer "worry" about safety involving the addict, there is reduced tension in the home, and there may even be gratitude that "something worse" is wrong.
A	Anger	This feeling is very individual. People have different awareness levels and modes of expression with anger. It can be an overt and strong feeling that is recognized by the significant other and readily expressed. On the other end of the spectrum is the person who feels displaced anger toward others and sees the addict as a victim. Or anger is an unacceptable feeling and the individual complains about physical ailments, idiosyncrasies of the program or denies having any feelings at all.
F	Fear	Fear is almost always about the future. Significant others fear relapse, worry about their financial future, and the effect the disease has had on their relationship, children, colleagues, extended family and friends.

(continued)

T	Tolerance	In time, significant others learn to tolerate the diagnosis of chemical dependency in their loved one. This feeling can be misinterpreted as acceptance, but this is only the beginning of that journey. Tolerance can be defined as "readiness to allow others to believe or act as they judge best."
D	Disappointment	The significant other expects sobriety along with the absence of personality defects. When the addict returns home with personality unchanged, and new dedication to others outside the family unit (12-step program participants), the significant other feels disappointment. This is often confusing because they feel they should be grateful for sobriety.
R	Reality	The "recovering" family now realizes that life goes on.
A	Acceptance	12-step meetings, sponsors, and an increased emphasis on spirituality allow the family to reach a point of acceptance. Living with the disease of chemical dependency no longer has the impact it did in early recovery. More friends and family are privy to this information and the family members may even feel comfortable helping others with this disease.
G	Growth	The significant other experiences a thirst for more knowledge, an ability to focus on self, and a deep connection with others in their situation. Others describe these individuals as "peaceful" when they sit in recovery groups with them.

°It is important to note that the significant other can "plateau" at any time. This is often described as feeling "stuck." The individual may be unaware of this process and only able to convey feelings of frustration.

"The time period in which these feelings are experienced varies, but they usually occur within the first 4 months. This is a common phase, called the "honeymoon," which couples experience when the patient is initially discharged, and/or during the Relief phase for the significant other. it will disappear.

10

Dual Diagnosis

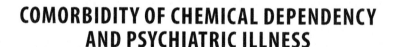

COMORBIDITY OF CHEMICAL DEPENDENCY AND PSYCHIATRIC ILLNESS

Addressed in this chapter are the highly complex processes of recognizing concomitant psychopathology in chemically dependent individuals. The existence of concomitant psychopathology with chemical dependencies, such as depression with alcoholism or character disorders with cocaine dependence, often presents diagnostic as well as treatment dilemmas.

Chemical dependency very often produces transitory mental status disturbances, which complicate this scenario, as does the recognition of addictive personality subtypes. The approach to these issues requires obtaining a very thorough patient history, including family history, mental status, exploration of intervals without chemical use, and premorbid history, as well as the need for careful collateral data from family and other treaters. Treatment considerations are complicated by the above mentioned factors, and the risks of some medication management strategies must be recognized. Risks also can include traditional individual or group psychotherapy targeting the psychiatric issues and not concentrating on the chemical dependency issues.

ADDICTIVE PERSONALITY: A HISTORICAL PERSPECTIVE

Over the years there has been speculation about a possible personality type common to all chemically dependent individuals. Years ago, a series of "trait studies" suggested that these addictive traits consisted primarily of a tendency toward depression and an antisocial personality structure (Weissman & Myers, 1980; Woodruff et al., 1973). Unfortunately, these populations were studied while they were actively using drugs or alcohol, during withdrawal, or in very early recovery. However, these trait studies seemed to forge an often skewed perception of chemically dependent people. It is difficult to determine whether traits are inherent in the alcoholic, for example, or consequences of the illness, particularly with the use of retrospective studies (Donovan, 1986). In the authors' experiences, the majority of altered affective states and personality characteristics, such as major depression or sociopathic behavior, are often an expression of the consequences of chemical dependency rather than any kind of premorbid pathology.

Behavioral tendencies, as well as a predisposition to certain anxieties and affective states, may certainly exist even prior to the use of any chemicals. This is consistent with the studies and observations that suggest a genetic as well as an early developmental link toward craving, and a neurochemical connection with mood-altering, addicting chemicals in those individuals with the disease of chemical dependency (see Chapter 1).

One series of neuropsychologic tests (Tarter et al., 1984) showed that the male offspring of chemically dependent parents (when compared with a control group), prior

to their ever using any chemicals, demonstrated a series of subtle but interesting tendencies. This subgroup showed evidence of an increase of childhood hyperactivity and problems with language processing. Also, evidence of deficiency in certain neurotransmitters in the prefrontal cortex, as well as alterations in evoked brain potentials, were suggested. Furthermore, Cloninger (1987), in his thesis on neurogenetic adaptive mechanisms in alcoholism, suggested that there are addictive personality traits with two specific subtypes. These subtypes involve specific neurotransmitters acting as neuromodulators. Neurotransmitter pathways may genetically determine craving and specific addictive personality traits. For example, stimulus hunger with type 2 alcoholism (late onset, binge pattern), according to Cloninger, utilizes dopamine as its neuromodulator.

Psychoanalytically oriented researchers, such as Khantzian (1985), have suggested that chemical use is based on the need to modify painful feeling states that predominate in the addiction-prone individual. This self-medication hypothesis (Khantzian, 1985) suggests that opiate use is a means of coping with feelings of rage, alcohol use a means of managing depression, and stimulant use an attempt to redirect the discomfort of an agitated depression, including the agitation that may come from a hypomanic state.

NARCISSISM AND ADDICTIVE PERSONALITY

The concept of narcissism is prevalent in analytic conceptions of addiction. Self psychology (Kohut, 1971) identifies narcissism as the result of deficits in early development. During early development, defects in nurturing by way of either neglect or abuse, produce significant deficits in ego strengths and self-esteem. Optimal frustration is critical to allow the child to eventually become autonomous from the parent and internalize the positive aspects of that parent. This is necessary for the development of strong ego strength, solid self-esteem, and the ability to be optimally soothed. In turn, a strong sense of self allows for an enhanced capacity to self-calm and self-soothe. If deficits are present, this capacity is diminished, necessitating outside elements (e.g., substance use and compulsive behaviors) to provide the self-calming or even self-energizing that comes from within. Furthermore, grandiosity is often used as a defense against deficits in self-esteem. Substance use can temporarily support this defensive grandiosity. However, this defense is fragile and invariably leads to increased dysphoria already increased by chronic substance abuse. The dysphoria fuels the need to obtain outside repair and, with the addict, substances are sought. A vicious cycle is set in motion: narcissistic deficits fuel the need for relief through chemicals because of the lack of self-regulatory capacity. The chemicals (along with defensive grandiosity) further diminish an already deficient sense of self, leading to further dysphoria and the need for more chemicals.

The analytic treatment approach would be to provide healthy self-object relations through interaction with the therapist, thereby strengthening self structures and reducing or eliminating the need for substance abuse. In part, this approach is like a more addiction oriented 12-step approach, which defines recovery as the ability to substitute meaningful, supportive relationships (meetings, sponsors, etc.) for chemicals. The expectation of complete abstinence in the initial phases of recovery, along with emphasis on the group process, can differentiate the addiction oriented approach from the analytic one. Also, the emphasis on a higher power in 12-step-oriented recovery further distinguishes these two approaches.

Twelve-Step-oriented concepts included, at times, references to problems with self-absorption. *The Twelve Steps and Twelve Traditions* (1953) discusses "ego puncturing," or the need to transcend the ego. In any case, the self psychology concept of narcissism provides important insights into an addictive personality style. Although research suggests that there is no single addictive personality style (Allen & Frances, 1986), we assert that chemical dependency includes a style of coping, along with certain tendencies toward emotions and behaviors that occur in addicts prior to the use of any mood-altering, addicting chemicals. The addictive personality style may then include a heightened level of anxiety, difficulties with delaying gratification (impulsiveness), and problems with self-esteem. At what point a definitive personality disorder (e.g., narcissistic) is differentiated from an addictive personality style is often difficult to assess.

One point of differentiation may be responsiveness to recovery. An addictive personality style typically responds dramatically to an addiction oriented treatment and 12-step recovery. A concomitant personality disorder may greatly interfere with one's capacity to substitute the human encounter (particularly in the group format) for the chemicals. Personality disorders, such as narcissistic personality disorder, are often characterized by individuals who perceive their problems as being totally external. This promotes feelings of victimization as well as denial. Lack of empathy and grandiosity would further prohibit the bonding necessary for recovery in these cases. Concomitant individual psychotherapy may be essential, along with a program of recovery to help facilitate the bonding process.

A narcissistic personality is "characterized by extreme self-centeredness and self-absorption, fantasies involving unrealistic goals, an excessive need for attention and admiration, and disturbed interpersonal relationships" (DSM, 1980). One of the more painful aspects of narcissism is a sense of loneliness (Kernberg, 1975). Narcissism in and of itself induces disturbances in feelings connected with others. This deficit in "relatedness" is essential to narcissistic states. The sense of aloneness or alienation is also descriptive of the isolation state found in addiction. Treating both narcissism and addiction depends on the process of emerging from isolation through connection with others.

PSYCHOLOGICAL PROFILE OF PHYSICIANS

A psychological profile specific to physicians, complicating an addictive personality style, has been suggested (Gabbard & Menninger, 1988). Physicians tend to be compulsive perfectionists (Gabbard, 1985). They also may use their profession as a means to defend against feelings of poor self-esteem that predated their becoming a physician and may have contributed to their choice of profession. Primary care physicians, in particular, receive the attention and nurturing from their patients that they did not get from their parents (Vaillant et al., 1972). The authors believe workaholism fits this pattern since it can be seen as an attempt to please an "internalized parent." Doubt, feelings of guilt, and a heightened sense of responsibility can exist in the physician's psychological profile. The profession itself fosters these feelings.

Considering that patients' lives and well-being hang in the balance, workaholism, compulsivity, and perfectionism are expected to some extent from physicians. Consequently, the fear of failure and its potential damage will foster self-doubt and feelings of guilt. To what extent the profession produces these tendencies or the tendencies themselves exist before entering the profession (and guide the individual into medicine) is an area of continued study. In any case, problems with self-esteem and self-doubt are considered part of the addictive personality overall. This may make the addicted physician more prone to a narcissistic style of functioning than the general addicted population. It certainly must be considered given the high percentage of narcissistic personality disorders in our outcome studies (see Chapter 2).

The tendency of physicians to be perfectionists and compulsive in their work can also be problematic in regards to addiction potential. The addicted physician typically justifies his addiction as a just reward for all his efforts. Often the physician rationalizes that his substance use has assisted him to put in longer hours and do more for patients.

The physician's need to control others is as potentially dangerous as any other factor (Gabbard & Menninger, 1988). Physicians can use the workplace as an environment that, under their control, will provide the nurturing and esteem they need. Feelings of omnipotence or the "M-Deity Syndrome" contribute to the addicted physician's enhanced denial and difficulty in self-observation. Cultural attitudes and expectations of placing the physician on a pedestal feed into these feelings of omnipotence.

PREVALENCE OF PSYCHIATRIC ILLNESS IN CHEMICALLY DEPENDENT PATIENTS

The literature regarding the prevalence of psychiatric illness among chemically dependent people is quite varied. Some estimate that 30 to 50% of all substance abusers who present for treatment have concomitant psychopathology, with affective disorder being most prominent (Rounsaville, Beissman, Crits-Christoph, Wilber, & Kleber, 1982). Researchers reviewing a range of studies found a 3 to 98% prevalence of depression among alcoholic patients (Keeler, Taylor, & Miller, 1979). This was dependent on whether the *Diagnostic and Statistical Manual of Mental Disorders* (DSM) criteria, Beck Depression Inventory, Schedule of Affective Disorder and Schizophrenia (SADS), or Research Diagnostic Criteria (RDC) were used in making the diagnosis of major depression. Many efforts have been made to determine the prevalence of psychiatric disorder in relation to a specific drug of choice. One study determined that 42% of all narcotic-dependent individuals had affective disorder when using SADS and RDC criteria, but only 9% when using DSM criteria and an unstructured interview (Rounsaville, Rosenberger, Wilber, Weissman, & Kleber, 1980).

Affective illness, particularly bipolar disorder, has been associated with cocaine dependence. Adult attention deficit disorder has been thought to be associated with stimulant dependence (including cocaine) (Weiss & Mirin, 1985). Other studies suggest that those individuals primarily addicted to depressants, such as alcohol, minor tranquilizers, or barbiturates, have an excessively high degree of panic and anxiety disorders (Mirin, Weiss, Michael, & Griffin, 1988). It has been observed that most alcoholics experience depressive symptoms secondary to their alcoholism, which usually disappear after a few weeks of abstinence, and that primary affective disorder with secondary alcoholism is much less frequent. Additionally, there is no clear genetic association between alcohol dependence and psychiatric illness (Shuckit, 1983). That is alcoholism and depression can be inherited, but depression and alcoholism as part of a depressive spectrum disease are not inherited together (Shuckit, 1986).

The variability in these studies suggests different possibilities. To begin with, different researchers have studied chemically dependent patients at variable times in their illness or recovery. The majority of studies have observed chemically dependent patients within only a few weeks of their abstinence. Also, many patients were observed in different settings, including treatment programs for chemical dependency, methadone maintenance settings, or even psychiatric settings. Clearly, the length of time in abstinence as well as quality of recovery are major factors in determining what degree of true comorbidity exists.

DIAGNOSING COMORBIDITY

One of the most important aspects of approaching comorbidity is to use extreme caution in avoiding premature diagnosis of psychiatric illness in chemical dependency. As suggested previously, multiple factors play a role in the demonstration of psychiatric symptomatology among chemically dependent patients.

The acute effects of the chemicals themselves, for instance, can give rise to multiple psychological impairments. For example, acute cocaine or stimulant intoxication can produce symptoms of paranoia or even thought disorder. The acute influence of alcohol or other sedative hypnotics on the central nervous system eventually produces depression in most individuals. Other chemicals such as opiates and marijuana can produce lethargy and anhedonia (reduced capacity to experience joy). Even beyond the acute effects of the chemical, chemical dependency is a clever imitator of psychiatric syndromes. Whether under the influence of the substance or withdrawal from the substance, psychological deficits are typically produced. Dependence on mood altering, addicting chemicals has dramatic effects on the human psyche. This disease produces significant regression, typically secondary to the isolation that occurs with chemical dependency, but also because of the erosion of healthy defense mechanisms. Healthy defense mechanisms, such as sublimation (the ability to rechannel frustration into energy), give way to more narcissistic defenses, such as blaming or projection. The combined effect of such deterioration characteristically produces an exaggeration of a person's character style or tendencies.

Therefore, if one has a tendency toward dysthymia, chemical dependency eventually will produce dysthymia and other symptoms concomitant with major depression. An individual with narcissistic deficits may develop a full-blown narcissistic personality disorder; borderline features may be exaggerated in chemical dependency. Even in premorbidly healthy individuals, the devastating effects of chemical dependency can induce an imitation of psychiatric illness that is simply a secondary, transient process.

The following case presents an example of comorbid conditions in a physician. It represents a composite of several actual cases.

Case 1

This 35-year-old male physician was admitted to his first psychiatric or alcohol and drug treatment program. The patient has a history of alcohol, amphetamine, and minor tranquilizer abuse through medical school. Following a back injury during his internship, he became dependent on codeine and propoxyphene, and this dependence persisted intermittently throughout his training. He self-treated the lethargy brought on by his pain medications with amphetamines and later cocaine. He suffered severe depression, and when attempting to reduce his use of chemicals, underwent trials on various tricyclic antidepressants combined with outpatient psychotherapy, with poor results.

He had no family history of endogenous depression or no personal history of severe endogenous depression prior to his drug use in late college and medical school. His cocaine abuse escalated despite numerous attempts to quit, and eventually he arrived at a program designed for chemically dependent health care professionals. He received a diagnosis of both chemical dependence and severe depression with vegetative features. The depression persisted for 3 months, despite treatment with a tetracyclic antidepressant and psychotherapy in addition to his program of recovery in the impaired professional's program. His own assumption was that he was endogenously depressed and that his cocaine and other addictions were secondary to this endogenous depression.

Discussion

After 3 months in the program, he stopped taking the antidepressants on his own and began to break through his denial system regarding chemical dependence. His depression steadily and completely receded as he more actively participated in the treatment program. He completed 5 months of treatment, including recovery residence living and mirror-image therapy. He is currently working as a physician, has been sober for more than 15 years, and has had no recurrence of depressive symptoms.

In this case, severe depression symptomatology persisted into the first several weeks of abstinence and involvement in a chemical dependency program. With time in the program and emphasis on recovery from chemical dependency, his symptoms of depression abated, suggesting that they were secondary phenomena (to the chemical dependency) rather than a concomitant primary disorder. This was further supported by no recurrence of symptoms of major depression over several years of abstinence and recovery. The final diagnosis for this patient: opiate and minor tranquilizer dependency; narcissistic personality traits.

THE NEED FOR CAUTION

A number of chemically dependent physicians, even those free of chemical use and in solid recovery, present with psychiatric illness. A painstaking effort must be made, however, not to diagnose a psychiatric illness prematurely, as this may lead to unnecessary medication and divert individuals from their efforts to prioritize their recovery from the chemical dependency.

For the purpose of diagnostic accuracy in determining comorbidity, nothing replaces a thorough personal and family history. Critical in taking the history of a chemical dependent individual is determining substances used, consequences of use, maladaptive behaviors, affective states, and existence of thought or perceptual disturbances.

A careful history of psychiatric symptoms should include a time frame indicating when the symptoms first occurred, whether the patient was under the influence of any chemicals or whether they occurred before initial use. Also, periods of protracted abstinence, especially periods of recovery where there was existence and continuation of psychiatric symptoms, are important to note. Again, one needs to consider that addictive personality traits often are exhibited well before the use of any mood-altering, addictive chemicals. Collateral data are essential in any history, particularly in this situation. Information gained not only from the patient but also from family members, significant others, and existing hospital or medical records are all critical in piecing together this difficult puzzle.

A careful physical evaluation is also essential. As we know, numerous psychiatric presentations can be precipitated by physical problems. For example, physical evidence of thyroid disease or neurologic dysfunction are two of the many kinds of physical abnormalities that can point to a physical cause for a behavioral difficulty. Hyperthyroidism can produce severe anxiety, depression, or even psychosis. Certainly residual physical affects from chemical use (such as hepatomegaly as a consequence of prolonged alcohol consumption) can produce encephalopathy, leading to different psychiatric presentations. Examples include organic affective syndrome or confusional states.

It is critical to get routine laboratory data, such as a complete blood count, SMA20 serum analysis, urinalysis, and, in some cases, HIV testing. These tests are not only critical from a baseline standpoint, but can provide additional information for the history and physical examination regarding organic causes for psychiatric symptoms.

Personality inventories provide critical baseline data for chemically dependent individuals overall. Caution should be used in the timing of administration of this or any other psychological test. Exaggerated or altered results may occur closer to the use of the last chemical and during the withdrawal state. Neuropsychological testing is critical, particularly when some degree of organic dysfunction is suspected, even after a period of time in recovery. In cases involving health care providers and other highly accountable individuals, this becomes even more critical because of the accountability factor. Projective testing can be particularly useful when trying to determine whether, or to what degree, character pathology exists in the chemically dependent individual.

The authors suggest that there be a period of time (i.e., 90 days) of complete abstinence before a definitive diagnosis of chemical dependency and concomitant psychiatric illness is made. However, abstinence alone for this period of time is not as critical as abstinence in a recovery setting. Abstinence is simply the absence of chemical use. Recovery is the replacement of chemical use with nonchemical coping skills, and the replacement of isolation with bonding with other individuals. Abstinence without recovery can prolong the imitation effect described earlier.

TREATING COMORBIDITY

Just as the most critical element in the diagnostic process is time in recovery, the same holds true for the initial approach to treatment in this population. In many cases, the best early treatment in the presence of psychiatric symptoms is taking a wait-and-see approach while maintaining the individual over a protracted period of time in abstinence and in a recovery process. Obviously, however, this is often a luxury clinicians do not have.

When psychiatric symptoms such as depression or anxiety or, in extreme cases, psychotic symptoms, clearly interfere with the individual's ability to remain in a recovery environment, every effort must be made to treat interfering symptoms aggressively. Too often those who treat chemically dependent patients are not aggressive enough in attempting to maintain this comorbid population in a recovery setting. The optimal treatment for any chemically dependent person, regardless of comorbid issues, involves an intensive treatment setting. In the past, we have feared that for patients lost to traditional psychiatry, the emphasis on treatment of chemical dependency would be lost or even ignored, or replaced by enabling types of treatment. Thus, it is important to bring psychiatric expertise to the chemical dependency setting to treat as many of these difficult patients as possible. However, some patients do need a brief stabilization in a psychiatric setting before spending time in a chemical dependency treatment setting.

The patient and significant others must be provided with in-depth explanations regarding the coexisting conditions and the rationale for the approaches taken. These issues should not be hidden, but clearly explained in the therapeutic community as well as in the small-group process. We approach these issues as an important aspect of an individual's recovery, just as we do any other such situations, medical, social, or otherwise.

Careful ongoing assessment of suicidal or homicidal potential also must be made. The literature indicates that both suicidal and homicidal potential is increased in chemically dependent individuals, whether dual diagnosis exists or not. This is further increased in the population with a dual diagnosis. Chemically dependent physicians with concomitant depression represent a very high suicide risk (Sargeant, Bruce, Florio, & Weissman, 1990).

Psychiatric symptoms must be treated aggressively, particularly in patients at high risk for psychiatric illness. Medication management, individual and group psychotherapy, and even electroconvulsive therapy may need to be combined with aggressive chemical dependency treatment for patients with a dual diagnosis. Medications must be used with caution in the chemically dependent population.

RISK FACTORS OF COMORBIDITY

The risks of pharmacotherapy and psychotherapy in a patient with suspected dual diagnosis include the following:

1. The patient may not really need it. Symptoms may represent a "dry drunk" phenomenon, i.e., a secondary effect of the chemical dependency.

2. Psychiatric intervention can make the situation worse by enhancing denial and preventing complete immersion in the chemical dependency program. Also, giving drugs to an addict at any time has inherent dangers.

3. Patients with a dual diagnosis, as well as those suffering from secondary psychiatric symptoms, often get better by working a program of recovery.

There are also risks in *not* treating psychiatrically. Neglecting to treat manageable psychopathology is comparable to withholding insulin from an insulin dependent diabetic. Withholding aggressive psychiatric treatment when indicated prevents an individual from receiving optimal treatment and care.

The ideal treatment for patients with a dual diagnosis includes the combined efforts of addiction treatment and psychiatry in a team approach. The addiction treatment should involve a solid understanding of psychopathology and would benefit from a psychiatric team that truly understands not only chemical dependency but also the process of recovery.

ADDITIONAL CASE STUDIES

The following cases are based on composites of individuals that we have seen over the years. Each case description is followed by a discussion in terms of an overall approach to the patient, additional data that later came to light, and the outcome of the case.

Case 2

This 37-year-old female family practitioner presented to our outpatient alcohol and drug program for an assessment of severe anxiety and panic attacks. She said that she had been sober and in the AA program for 7 years. Her involvement is very active, chairing meetings, and often sponsoring a number of different people. She described her panic as being an intermittent problem throughout her adult life, but particularly increasing over the past 2 years. She said that her panic does not seem to be precipitated by any particular event. She described panic attacks that seem to last 10 minutes to a half-hour and occur anywhere from once or twice a week. She said that they often occur when she is driving her car or seeing patients. She described a sense of impending doom, pounding in her chest, feeling flushed, numb lips, tingling in her hands, diaphoresis, and lightheadedness. She had been extremely reluctant to seek professional help for this problem because of unsatisfactory treatment from past physicians and psychiatrists. She also feared being put on medications that might interfere with her recovery from alcoholism. These attacks eventually had become so severe and debilitating that she felt she needed to seek some kind of professional assistance.

Discussion

In this case, significant symptoms of anxiety and panic occurred after a considerable period of time in what appears to be a solid recovery. Further analysis showed a history of panic attacks when the patient was in her late twenties, occurring about the time of her alcohol abuse. Additionally, a family history revealed that her mother was alcoholic and depressed. The mother was hospitalized for one year when the patient was 9 years old. Also, the patient had been divorced for 4 years. These additional data are particularly important. The history of separation during the patient's youth (and a more recent history of divorce) brings up abandonment issues, which have been suggested as part of the dynamics of patients with anxiety and panic disorders. A careful workup ruled out organic causes, including hyperthyroidism, pheochromocytoma, and complex partial seizures. The patient was considered for either a selective serotonin reuptake inhibitor or imipramine regimen along with supportive psychotherapy. Imipramine therapy was tried first, but she did not respond; however, she did respond to a selective serotonin reuptake inhibitor. The patient did well.

Not only was there relief from the considerable painful symptoms of panic disorder, but possible relapse of her alcoholism precipitated by the panic was avoided, as was continued interference with her practice. This patient's final diagnosis was: alcohol dependence in remission and panic disorder.

Case 3

This 34-year-old physician (psychiatrist) was admitted to an inpatient chemical dependency unit following an acute episode of depression, anxiety, and paranoia. He had been admitted 3 years earlier to an inpatient alcohol and drug treatment program following at least 7 years of severe multi-substance abuse. These substances included alcohol and diazepam.

The patient was extremely depressed on this admission and became increasingly so during his stay. After 2 weeks on the unit, he became suicidal and was transferred to a general psychiatric unit elsewhere in that hospital. On his transfer, he was diagnosed as having an agitated depression and was placed on both amitriptyline and alprazolam. He seemed to have some degree of response and after 3 weeks was discharged under the care of the psychiatrist who followed him after the transfer. The patient remained on amitriptyline and alprazolam following his discharge and underwent weekly individual psychotherapy. His alcohol and drug use declined, but he drank occasionally and intermittently used cocaine on a "social" basis. Both the patient and his psychiatrist felt that the major problem was depression, which, they said, explained his response to the amitriptyline and alprazolam.

Two months later, the patient stopped seeing his psychiatrist and also refrained from taking his medication. After ceasing the medication, he began experiencing anxiety and then depression with a strong element of agitation and paranoia. He began using cocaine and alcohol to a greater extent. He also started using alprazolam again on his own. The patient contacted his psychiatrist again, which led to another admission to a psychiatric unit.

Discussion

This individual gave a history consistent with depression, coexisting anxiety, and significant chemical abuse and dependence. However, the patient had primarily received psychiatric treatment. Chemical dependency treatment had been aborted by a transfer to a psychiatric unit following his suicidal ideation, consequently, it was not prioritized. This is evidenced by the use of alprazolam along with an antidepressant (not establishing total abstinence from mood altering, addicting chemicals), and not utilizing the support of a recovery program.

Further evidence in the family history revealed that the patient's father was alcoholic, hospitalized for depression, and was a suicide. It was also revealed that the patient had experienced severe depression before he was 18 years old and did not seek professional intervention. This was a year prior to the use of any mood-altering, addicting chemicals.

The patient was eventually transferred to an alcohol and drug treatment center after detoxification. He was maintained on amitriptyline since a concomitant depression was clinically evident and supported by his personal and family history. The alprazolam therapy was stopped. He eventually went to an extended-care program that specialized in treating health care professionals. Following the specialized program, he was taken off amitriptyline. After several weeks his depression rapidly returned with the previous intensity. Amitriptyline therapy was restarted.

From a long-term treatment program, he went into an extended halfway house. The amitriptyline was eventually tapered off after a year. He had a recurrence of depression 2 years later and responded to amitriptyline. He has remained sober for 4 years.

In this case, withholding antidepressant therapy after a period in recovery demonstrated true concomitant psychiat-

ric illness, i.e., depression. With more data currently available, it appears that maintenance doses of amitriptyline may have prevented the recurrences of depression.

Since this patient was himself a physician, more specifically a psychiatrist, he had been able to manipulate his care and essentially take control of his treatment for years. In essence, he was self-diagnosing and self-treating, which is typical for the chemically dependent physician. Participation in an extended specialty program for health care professionals assisted him in adapting to his role as a patient. This patient's final diagnosis: chemical dependency and major depression, recurrent.

SUMMARY

Dual diagnosis or comorbidity of chemical dependency and psychiatric illness presents many challenges. Thorough diagnostic approaches must include allowing enough time in true recovery before final conclusions are made. Treatment must be aggressive and optimally involve a team including both psychiatric- and addiction-medicine components. Medication management and psychotherapeutic techniques should be used with utmost care and discretion in this population. If the correct approaches are used, this population can be effectively treated and obtain maximum benefit.

11

Legal Considerations for the Chemically Dependent Physician

This chapter will discuss legal issues regarding chemical dependency and impairment. The legal definition of impairment, interface with regulatory services, and support systems also are explored. An overview of the characteristics and problems unique to physicians, including prevention, intervention, treatment, and continuing care, precede the discussion of legal aspects.

"Troubled physicians" have been described as those who are incompetent due to a lack of skill or knowledge or to an impairment arising from a physical or mental disorder, including chemical dependency. The "sick doctor statute" defines the inability to practice medicine with reasonable skill and safety to his patients because of one or more enumerable illnesses (American Medical Association, Council on Mental Health, 1973).

If a physician exhibits compulsive use of one or more mood-altering, addicting chemicals for a period of time, demonstrating interference with his or her practice or in other areas of life, it is easy to recognize the need for intervention, treatment, and aftercare monitoring. Those of us who provide treatment programs for physicians recognize that there are special circumstances (described below) regarding this chemically dependent population.

It can be particularly difficult to get physicians into treatment simply because they have trouble seeing their own problems. After years of training and practice, they can begin to feel as though they have few or no faults. They become so immersed in their roles as "healers" and "authority figures" that the ability for introspection can become increasingly impaired. Although physicians are often described as arrogant, this may be less the issue than the need to feel worthy of his patients' respect and trust.

Physicians become experts in diagnosing disease in other human beings, and many also see themselves as experts in self-diagnosis. When a disease process as sensitive as chemical dependency is involved, the physician may misdiagnose his or her own symptoms.

Considering the number of years involved in obtaining a license to practice medicine, the investment of self-esteem, and the financial sacrifices typically made, physicians and, very often, their families are extremely defensive about any intervention that may pose a threat to that license or to the ability to practice medicine. Despite the many reassurances we can give to the physician and the family, identification and treatment of chemical dependency is still perceived as a threat.

Physicians clearly have greater access to controlled substances than the general population, given the opportunities for self-prescribing, obtaining professional samples, or taking advantage of the easy availability of substances in the office or hospital setting. It is, in fact, often unusual prescribing practices, traced by state licensing boards through triplicate forms or other means, that bring the physician to the attention of disciplinary bodies.

Physicians are licensed to provide competent and satisfactory patient care. As occurs with many diseases, chemical dependency eventually interferes with this ability. Obtaining medical help and rehabilitation for his or her disease is a right, as it is for any individual. But reentry into the medical profession is a privilege. For such rehabilitation and reentry to occur appropriately for the well-being of patients, certain guidelines specific to physicians must be observed in treatment and aftercare monitoring.

PREVENTION

With the growing awareness of chemical dependency as a disease, state medical societies have formed impaired physician committees, as well as hospital based committees, which have been active in the prevention of chemical dependency. This prevention is most facilitated by acknowledging the risk factors (Talbott, 1984), as well as by clearly communicating the disease concept of chemical dependency to the public.

State medical society impaired physician committees are now more generally termed physician health committees, and they usually have a membership who either have personal experience with chemical dependency and are themselves recovering or are familiar with the disease and may have a good deal of empathy and caring for those who suffer from it. Part of the function of these committees is to educate the general public and the medical community about the chemically dependent physician. Community lectures help to designate the addiction as a disease and to communicate that physicians with this disease will be supported for rehabilitation and reentry. Nurses, dentists, and pharmacists have similar advocacy groups.

In addition, hospital based committees, often called wellness committees, are being set Up throughout the country. These committees are independent from hospital disciplinary committees, and their purpose, like that of the state medical societies' committees, is to act as advocates for the impaired physician. These committees often provide educational information to the various departments throughout the hospital in which they are based, and also extend that information to the physicians' families. These committees typically have reinforced health and fitness as a means of minimizing stress in a hospital practice. For example, "fun runs" that involve physicians, their families, and other personnel in jogging or other athletic competitions have been used as a means of both education and prevention.

Intervention (Talbott & Cooney, 1982) can occur on many levels, and state or hospital based committees are es- sential in facilitating it. In general, intervention should not be attempted by one individual, and, of course, it should always be done in good faith. The ideal intervention (Tal- bott & Cooney, 1982) includes as many individuals as can be gathered to confront the impaired physician. This may include the spouse, other family members, the individual's partner, or concerned nurses, in addition to members of the hospital or state based committee. An intervention team, consisting of two or more individuals trained in dealing with chemical dependency, should coordinate the intervention.

A physician is seldom willing at first to go into treatment. Generally, the physician's response to an intervention is one of anger, shame, and embarrassment. Additional methods are then necessary to get the individual into treatment. The disciplinary committee of the hospital or the state medical society may need to threaten the physician with a loss of privileges (and ultimately with the loss of his or her license) for an intervention to be completely successful. Such threats are a last resort, but unfortunately often become necessary. Usually the threat of reporting the physician's impairment to the hospital disciplinary committee is successful without having to go any further.

Case 1

A 63-year-old obstetrician had been struggling with alcohol dependency for several years. His wife called the hotline of the state medical society physicians assistance program. The medical director of the state medical society received the information from the wife, which included the physician's 7-year history of progressive daily drinking. Related behavior included blackouts, mood swings, and increased agitation. The wife stated that her husband had generally kept his drinking separate from his work, but that he recently had had to cancel surgeries and outpatient visits. The physician's partner in his practice, as well as some of his office staff, had expressed concern. His wife further stated that previous attempts at trying to get her husband into treatment had failed.

Investigation by the state medical society confirmed his wife's story and indicated that several office staff, as well as his partner, were concerned about the physician's drinking and the progression of the disease process. Additionally, reports had been made to the physicians' assistance committee at the hospital; this committee also expressed concern about the physician. There was no indication that any information had been given to the hospital disciplinary committee, nor had any disciplinary action been taken by the hospital.

An intervention was arranged that included two of the physician's office personnel. One was his primary partner in the practice, and the other was one of the members of the physicians' assistance committee of the hospital. The intervention was directed by the medical director of the state medical society. When confronted, the physician became quite angry and defensive. Several attempts were made to empathize with and support him. The intervention team insisted on an assessment at a treatment center that dealt with health care professionals. The physician initially refused. The medical director stated that, considering the progression of the alcoholism and the concerns that had already been shared, refusal to follow through on the recommendations would necessitate presenting his case to the disciplinary committee of the hospital. It was only at this point that the physician agreed to an assessment at a treatment center. The assessment concluded that he suffered from progressive alcoholism and would benefit from treatment.

Here, as in so many cases, the threat of being reported was enough to encourage compliance with the recommendations that were made. Very few such interventions are unsuccessful, with the physician being determined to remain chemically dependent and ultimately refusing treatment. If the physician does refuse to comply, however, any disciplinary action involving his hospital privileges must be reported to the state licensing board by the hospital.

TREATMENT

Recognizing the complex issues regarding chemically dependent physicians, several treatment programs that provide specialized care for health care professionals have been developed (see Chapter 2). Initially, as previously indicated, there must be a thorough assessment by a multidisciplinary team. The assessment team then presents the physician and his or her family with a diagnosis and treatment options. If chemical dependency treatment is indicated, then at least three facilities are given as options. The first treatment phase is often a combination of inpatient and intensive outpatient treatment, usually involving a residential setting. This is followed by mirror-image placement therapy, in which the physician is a patient while assuming some responsibilities as a professional within the treatment setting (Talbott, 1984). The placement phase offers impaired physicians practice in caring for other individuals while also caring for themselves and prioritizing their recovery in a practical situation.

CONTINUING CARE

Another major component of treatment is extended aftercare. The specialized programs throughout the country understand that physicians need to be with their peers to break through the sense of uniqueness that often imposes a struggle while they are in treatment. This peer setting allows for a degree of confrontation as well as the support essential for effective treatment. Issues regarding liability, licensure, hospital privileges, and so on are somewhat unique to the chemically dependent physician, and the presence of peers in treatment groups provides understanding and support in these difficult areas.

Aftercare is one of the most important elements in treating the impaired physician. A specialized treatment program for physicians generally involves a minimum of 20 months of continuing care. This monitoring includes weekly meetings of professionally facilitated monitoring groups and random urine monitoring, as well as individual sessions with the primary physician (typically a physician on staff at the treatment facility). The treatment program will further establish a contact person at the practice site for the physician. This may be the head of a particular department or a peer in the private practice setting. In any case, this contact person should have a direct line of communication to the primary physician of the monitoring treatment program.

The aftercare monitoring system is best implemented with a contingency contract. This written contract also may involve the state medical society's impaired physicians committee, and even the state licensing board if the board was involved with the patient prior to treatment. A 12-step recovery program such as AA is also considered essential in maintaining sobriety and is a prioritized expectation in the aftercare contract. Violation of the treatment contract, such as failure to attend required group meetings or relapse, will be dealt with on an individual basis with clear-cut relapse guidelines (Talbott & Martin, 1984). Some action will be taken, possibly including a readjustment of the practice setting and/or further treatment in some modified form.

All involved in aftercare must understand that, if there is a breach of the contract and an unwillingness by the patient to follow treatment recommendations, the situation will usually be communicated to the contact person at the participating practice site. At this point, the contact person may be responsible for reporting the situation to a disciplinary body. This would only occur under the most extreme circumstances, in which the physician may pose a threat to patient care.

Case 2

A 49-year-old anesthesiologist completed a specialized longterm treatment program for fentanyl (a powerful opiate used in anesthesia) dependency. This physician was admitted to the facility for what had progressed to daily use of intravenous fentanyl. A successful intervention took place, and the physician entered a long-term specialized treatment program for physicians. The physician successfully completed 4 months of treatment and returned to his practice of anesthesiology. He was not only involved in the typical aftercare contract, but was also placed on naltrexone, an opiate antagonist that would further deter any use of opiates. Urine samples were obtained to test for both fentanyl and naltrexone in addition to the regular aftercare contract.

The physician did very well for 6 months, but then stopped taking the naltrexone for a few days and began taking fentanyl. This was caught almost immediately by aftercare monitoring. The physician was placed back into the treatment setting for a 3-week evaluation of the process. It became clear during this brief treatment interlude and review of the relapse that, despite the successful completion of treatment and the in-depth aftercare monitoring, the return to anesthesiology was not consistent with recovery. The pressures and circumstances of this practice placed the patient at too great a risk, despite the best efforts and intentions. The patient agreed to pursue a specialty in psychiatry, where exposure to narcotics and other high-risk issues would be minimized.

LEGAL ASPECTS

Confidentiality and danger are major issues in the treatment of chemically dependent physicians. Confidentiality involves a therapeutic setting where the patient and therapist can enter a relationship based on trust. Confidentiality in psychiatric treatment is considered an ethical obligation, based both on the Hippocratic oath and the American Psychiatric Association (1978) principles of medical ethics with special annotations applicable to psychiatry. Confidentiality is enforced by law, but this protection has been eroding over the past 10 years, primarily in cases where a patient is deemed dangerous either to self or others. Recent case law, starting with Tarasoff v. Regents of the University of California (1974, 1976), indicates that when a patient is foreseeably dangerous to another person, the therapist can, and in some cases must, breach the confidentiality of the doctor — patient relationship to protect the third party.

The treatment of a chemically dependent physician is problematic for the treating physician. Because of the issue of danger to the impaired physician's patients, the question of agency arises. Is the treating physician an agent of the patient solely, or automatically also an agent of society for monitoring other physicians? There are cogent arguments for both the need for absolute confidentiality, and the required reporting of information involving the incompetence of other physicians. Court decisions in malpractice cases indicate that physicians and hospital staff who know or should have known of patient care compromised by an impaired health care professional can and often will be held liable for any harm that may arise.

In addition to the ethical guidelines and relevant case law, other regulatory and monitoring agencies focus attention on the impaired physician. As mentioned earlier, every state medical society (and many hospitals) now have some committee that focuses on identification of the early intervention for the impaired physician. The intervention and monitoring programs of the state medical societies are either noncoercive, in which there is no reporting to the state medical board, or coercive, in which noncompliance or danger to patients may be reported. Every state also has a medical practice act, the provisions of which are frequently violated by chemically dependent physicians, particularly with regard to prescribing regulations. The medical practice act is enforced by a state medical board and a state licensing board.

The legal department of the American Medical Association (AMA) created a model impaired physician treatment act that enhances the role of the state medical societies and their treatment programs. More than 30 states have adopted this model legislation, while others have drawn from it (AMA, 1988). Today, more than 40 states have granted licensing boards or medical societies the express authority to investigate and provide rehabilitation with varying degrees of confidentiality as an alternative to punitive law.

REPORTING

By 1980, at least 39 states had enacted some form of a "sick doctor" statute. The requirements for reporting an impaired

physician vary considerably from state to state. Some of these states allow reporting and others mandate it. Immunity for good-faith reporting is usually included in the statute. Reports are generally made to the state medical licensing board.

Reporting has been aided by the formation of a National Practitioner Data Bank for Adverse Information on Physicians and Other Health Care Practitioners. Entrance into a drug, alcohol, and psychiatric rehabilitation program does not in and of itself constitute a reportable action. For example, if the physician voluntarily enters a program and the hospital offers him a leave of absence, this is not reportable. However, involuntary entrance into a program is reportable if a physician refuses to enter after being judged as having a condition that affects competence or conduct, with restrictions imposed on his clinical privileges for more than 30 days. Entry is also reportable if an express agreement is made to relinquish or restrict a physician's privileges in return for the hospital not conducting an investigation of possible incompetence or improper professional conduct when there is evidence of substance abuse.

The situation is different when the state medical society, hospital, or licensing board is not involved and the physician seeks treatment under some other conditions (e.g., voluntarily). Unless the treating physician, as a condition of treatment, has the impaired physician sign a release allowing communication with a disciplinary body, he may be bound by the confidentiality law. Many, but not all, state statutes allow breaches of doctor–patient confidentiality when patients are assessed as dangerous to self or others.

The reporting physician or group must act in good faith when reporting. Hospitals have a duty to provide competent and satisfactory patient care, and the hospital staff has a responsibility to monitor physicians' performance (Busch, 1985). The legal doctrine *respondent superior* maintains that a hospital may be liable for the negligent acts of any employee when those acts are committed within the employee's duties and obligations in that hospital setting. Whenever impairment is identified in a hospital setting, noncoercive intervention is recommended to encourage the physician to seek treatment (Webster, 1983).

Newer means to resolve disputes between impaired practitioners and hospitals that involve reporting to state and national bodies include mediation (which is not binding) and arbitration (which is binding). This is often a two-step process. The advantages are that no public record is generated and public disclosures concerning the proceedings generally are not made unless by action of one of the parties. These means of resolution permit the hospital and the physician to resolve disputes privately, without the fear of public scrutiny. However, the threat of reporting still may be needed to encourage the physician to enter treatment.

When an impaired physician refuses help and staff privileges are restricted or denied, the hospital has the responsibility to notify the state licensing board. The state licensing board then will investigate and usually continue attempts to get the physician into treatment. The licensing board will schedule a hearing, and if impairment is documented, treatment will often be a condition for licensure. The board has the ability to suspend or revoke licensure, as well as put a license on probationary status, depending on the outcome of the rehabilitation process.

In our experience at Rush and Talbott, the licensing boards have been supportive in cases involving chemical dependency. The licensing board expects that appropriate treatment will be completed and that an aftercare monitoring contract will be successfully followed. Licensure has generally been maintained and supported in such cases. Currently, licensing boards in many states query physicians only about their present state of health and do not inquire about previous disease or treatment.

DISABILITY AND POTENTIAL DISCRIMINATION

Despite outstanding recovery rates among appropriately treated and monitored physicians, there has been an unfortunate.. growing tendency for discrimination. In the last few years, some third-party payers have eliminated physicians who have an agreement with the state licensing board from being providers. This has occurred even when physicians have voluntarily contacted the licensing board for an informal agreement. In some cases, third-party providers have used this kind of licensure encumberment to eliminate recovering physicians. This is particularly disconcerting because licensing boards are intended to be part of a system that helps to provide better monitoring and outcomes in recovery. The majority of consent orders or licensure agreements should not restrict the recovering physician from full practice, but provide guidelines to ensure better compliance with a recovery program.

The same discrimination has been seen in some of the specialty boards. Some have gone so far as to revoke board certification based on information regarding impaired physicians. Others have reasonably prolonged the period of time that someone can sit for the licensing examination following treatment for chemical dependency (e.g., 1 to 2 years of sobriety required).

There is a growing body of evidence (see Chapter 2) that recovery rates are excellent when impaired physicians are properly treated and monitored. It is hoped that this will help to deter the problem of discrimination against these physicians. The Americans with Disabilities Act (ADA) of 1990 (a law that became effective in 1992) also may help fight these kinds of discriminatory practices. This law applies to persons who have complied with a recognized treatment program for substance abuse and who either wish to return to their former employment or are seeking new employment. The ADA prohibits discrimination in employment practices, such as hiring, compensation, and firing, and requires employers to hire workers with disabilities if, were he or she without the disability, the worker is the best-qualified individual. In other words, a qualified individual with a disability who can perform the essential functions of a job without accommodation or with "reasonable accommodation" must be given the same opportunity to be hired or retained as an individual without a disability.

Other entities are taking action against these discriminatory practices as well. At the AMA House of Delegate's annual meeting in 1992, a resolution was adopted regarding discrimination against physicians under the supervision of a medical examining board. The resolution stated that the AMA opposed the exclusion of otherwise capable physicians from employment, business opportunity, insurance coverage, specialty board certification or recertification, and other benefits, solely because he or she is or has been under the supervision of a medical licensing board (a consent order requiring compliance with an aftercare contract) in a program of rehabilitation.

Also in 1992, a report from the Committee on Alcoholism of the Medical Society of New York stated concerns regarding the growing number of licensing, certifying, and other agencies requiring applicants to answer questions about their history of referral and treatment for alcohol and drug disorders and mental and emotional illness. A formal request was made to the Medical Society to replace such questions with those regarding an applicant's current ability to practice medicine. The American Society of Addiction Medicine, through their Committee for Physician's Health, is compiling documentation for a position paper to help educate these agencies regarding the need to support recovering physicians and the dangers of not doing so. It is also organizing a list of firms and attorneys experienced in physician discrimination.

Growing discrimination will only reverse the significant progress made over the last several years in the treatment, reentry, and support of the recovering physician. If this problem continues to grow, it will produce an environment in which punitive action is the rule, driving the problem of chemical dependency and impairment back underground. In turn, this will produce more impairment problems, and physicians and their families, as well as patient care, will suffer. It is the intent and duty of the authors and others (i.e., International Doctors in Alcoholics Anonymous and the American Society of Addiction Medicine) to fight this type of discrimination.

COERCION INTO TREATMENT

The successful rehabilitation of a chemically dependent physician depends in part on the ability of the treating professionals and treatment program to act as advocates and fully support the physician's rehabilitation and reentry into the medical profession.

Trust is also an essential element for a successful treatment outcome in any therapeutic situation. Because of denial and fear of consequences, most physicians enter treatment as a result of some degree of coercion. That coercion may come from a disciplinary body, such as a hospital, state medical society, or licensing board, or from partners or family members. In any case, a minority of impaired physicians come into treatment completely of their own volition.

Coercion is not always a negative influence. Realistically, even the impaired physician who enters treatment willingly and has totally surrendered to his need for help (Deitch & Zweben, 1984) has experienced a form of coercion from the disease itself. Chemical dependency forces an individual to suffer significantly through a series of losses (both financial and interpersonal), and ultimately through loss of control associated with drug use. In this way, the greatest degree of coercion really comes from the disease process. Complete surrender to the treatment process is essential for long-term recovery. Coercion, both from the law and from the disease, can clearly act as an impetus.

In some situations, impaired physicians who enter treatment because of coercion (from the licensing board, family, and so on) remain quite angry and distrustful. Such unabated anger may be a symptom of continued resistance to treatment. Remaining resentment and anger regarding the coercion, despite continued treatment, may portend a reduced likelihood of long-term recovery, and must be considered in treatment planning.

Usually, however, coercion into treatment becomes less of an issue once the recovery process begins. Ultimately, it may even be viewed as a gift, since it brought the impaired physician into the treatment process that will likely improve the quality of his life. Many monitored physicians in both the Rush and Talbott programs request continued monitoring as it presents a positive, measurable marker of their chemical sobriety.

References

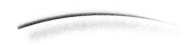

Alcoholics Anonymous, World Services, Inc. (1953). *The twelve steps and twelve traditions.* New York: Author.

Alcoholics Anonymous, World Services, Inc. (1976). *Alcoholics Anonymous* (3rd ed.). New York: Author.

Allen, M. H., & Frances, R. J. (1986). Varieties of psychopathology found in patients with addictive disorders: A review. In R. E. Meyer (Ed.), *Psychopathology and addictive disorders* (pp. 17-38). New York: Guilford Press.

American Medical Association (AMA). (1986). AMA *Women in medicine project.* Chicago: Author.

American Medical Association (AMA). (1988). *Summary of activities, impaired physician program.* Chicago: Author.

American Medical Association, Council on Mental Health. (1973). The sick physician: Impairment of psychiatric disorder including alcoholism and drug dependence. *Journal of the American Medical Association, 223,* 684-687.

American Psychiatric Association. (1978). *Principles of medical ethics with annotations especially applicable to psychiatry.* Washington, DC: American Psychiatric Press.

American Psychiatric Association. (1980). *Diagnostic and statistical manual of mental disorders* (3rd ed.). Washington, DC: American Psychiatric Press.

American Psychiatric Association. (1987). *Diagnostic and statistical manual of mental disorders* (3rd ed. rev.) . Washington, DC: American Psychiatric Press.

Angres, D. H., & Benson, W. H. (1985). Cocainism: A workable model for recovery. *Psychiatric Medicine, 3*(4), 369-388.

Angres, D., & Busch, K. (1989). The chemically dependent physician: Clinical and legal considerations. Legal implications of hospital policies and practices. In R. D. Mill (Ed.), *New directions in mental health services* (pp. 21-32). San Francisco: Jossey-Bass.

Beattie, M. (1989). *Beyond codependency and getting better all the time.* San Francisco: Harper and Row.

Bennett, G., & Woolf, D. S. (1983). Current approaches to substance abuse therapy. In G. Bennett, C. Vourakis, & D. S. Woolf (Eds.), *Substance abuse: Pharmacological, development, and clinical perspectives* (pp. 341-369). New York: Wiley.

Bickel, J. (1988). *Women in medicine statistics.* Washington, DC: Association of American Medical Colleges.

Bissell, L. (1984, August 15). *Plenary Address.* The 24th Southeastern School of Alcohol and Drug Studies. Athens: University of Georgia.

Bissell, L., & Haberman, P. (1984). *Alcoholism in the professions.* New York: Oxford University Press.

Bissell, L., & Jones, R. W. (1976). The alcoholic physician: A survey. *American Journal of Psychiatry, 133,* 1142-1146.

Bissell, L., & Skorina, J. K. (1987). One hundred alcoholic women in medicine. *Journal of the American Medical Association, 257,* 2939-2944.

Blachly, P. H., Disher, W., & Roduner, G. (1968, December). Suicide by physicians. *Bulletin of Suicide.*

Blondell, R. D. (1993). Impaired physicians. *Primary Care, 20,* 209-219.

Blum, K., Noble, E. P., Sheridan, P. J., Montgomery, A., Ritchie, T., Jagadeeswaran, P., Nogami, H., Brigg, A. H., & Cohn, J. B. (1990). Allelic association of human dopamine D2 receptor gene in alcoholism. *Journal of the American Medical Association, 263(15),* 2055-2060.

Blum, K., & Payne, J. (1991). The somatopsychic syndrome: A blueprint for behavior. *Addiction and Recovery, 11,* 4-5.

Blum, K., & Trachtenberg, M. (1987). Alcohol and opiod peptides: Neuropharmacological rationale for physical craving of alcohol. *American Journal of Drug and Alcohol Abuse, 13(3),* 365-372.

Busch, K. A. (1985). The impaired physician: Hospital/medical staff liability and due process of law. *Psychiatric Medicine, 2,* 262-271.

Canavan, D. (1984). Impaired physician: Hospital/medical staff liability and due process of law. *Psychiatric Medicine, 2,* 262-271. Canavan, D. (1984). Impaired physicians program, monitoring. *Journal of the Medical Society of New Jersey, 81,* 65-66.

Cloninger, C. R. (1987). Neurogenetic adaptive mechanisms in alcoholism. *Science, 236,* 410-416.

Coe, C. L., Glass, J. C., Weiner, S. G., & Levine, S. (1983). Behavioral, but not physiological, adaptation to repeated separation in mother and infant primates. *Psychoneuroendocrinology, 8,* 401-409.

Corrigan, E. M. (1980). *Alcoholic women in treatment.* New York: Oxford University Press.

Deitch, D., & Zweben, J. (1984) . Coercion in the therapeutic community. *Journal of Psychoactive Drugs, 16,* 35-41.

Dinwiddie, S., & Cloninger, C. R. (1991). Family and adoption studies in alcoholism and drug addiction. *Psychiatric Annals, 21,* 206-214.

Donovan, J. M. (1986). An etiologic model of alcoholism. *American Journal of Psychiatry, 143,* 1-11.

Faraj, B. A., Lenton, J. D., Kutner, M., Camp, V. M., Stammers, T. W., Lee, S. R., Lollies, P. A., Chandora, D. (1987). Prevalence of low monoamine oxidase function in alcoholism. *Alcoholism, Clinical & Experimental Research, 11(5),* 464-467.

Festinger, L. (1957). *A theory of cognitive dissonance.* Evanston, IL: Row, Peterson.

Fink, E. B., Longabaugh, R., McCrady, B., Stout, R. L., Beanie, M., Ruggierri-Authelet, A., & McNeil, D. (1985). Effectiveness of alcoholism treatment in partial versus inpatient settings: 24 month outcomes. *Addictive Behaviors, 10(3),* 235-248.

Finley, B. G. (1983). The family and substance abuse. In G. Bennett, C. Vourakis, & D. S. Woolfe (Eds.), *Substance abuse: Pharmacological, development, and clinical perspectives* (pp. 119-134). New York: Wiley.

Fluharty, D. G., Jr. (1996). Urine drug screening for health professionals. *Journal of Medical Licensure and Discipline, 83, 84:* 202-208.

Frolich, W. D. (1972). Alienation. In H. J. Eysenak (Ed.), *Encyclopedia of psychiatry.* New York: Herder & Herder.

Gabbard, G. 0. (1985). The role of compulsiveness in the normal physician. *Journal of the American Medical Association, 254,* 2926-2929.

Gabbard, G. 0. (1992). Psychodynamic psychiatry in the "decade

of the brain." *American Journal of Psychiatry, 149,* 991-998. Gabbard, G. 0., & Menninger, R. W. (1988). *Medical marriages.*

Washington, DC: American Psychiatric Press.

Gallegos, K., Lubin, B., Bowers, C., Blevins, J., Talbott, G. D., & Wilson, P. (1992, April). Relapse and recovery: 5-10 years follow-up study of chemically dependent physicians: The Georgia experience. *Maryland Medical Journal, 41,* 315-319.

Gallegos, K. V., & Norton, M. (1984). Characterization of Georgia's Impaired Physicians Program treatment population. *Journal of the Medical Association of Georgia, 74,* 755-758.

Gallegos, K. V., Veit, F. W., Wilson, P., Porter, T. L., & Talbott, G. D. (1988). Substance abuse among health professionals. *Maryland Medical Journal, 37(3),* 191-197.

Gardner, E. (1992). Brain reward mechanisms. In J. H. Lowinson, P. Ruiz, & R. B. Millman (Eds.), *Substance abuse: A comprehensive textbook* (2nd ed., pp. 73-75). Baltimore: Williams & Wilkins.

Giannini, A. J., & Miller, N. S. (1989). Drug abuse: A biopsychiatric model. *American Family Physician, 40(5)*, 173-182.

Gitlow, S. E. (1980). An overview. In S. E. Gitlow & H. S. Peyser (Eds.). *Alcoholism: A practical treatment guide* (pp. 263-294). New York: Grune & Stratton.

Goodwin, D., Schulsinger, F., Moller, N., Hermansen, L., Winokur, G., & Guze, S. B. (1974). Drinking problems in adopted and non-adopted sons of alcoholics. *Archives of General Psychiatry, 31*, 134-164.

Hoffman, N., Halikas, J., & Mee-Lee, D. (1996). Patient placement criteria for the treatment of psychoactive substance use disorders (2nd. ed.). Washington, DC: American Society of Addictive Medicine.

Jackson, J. (1954). The adjustment of the family to the crisis of alcoholism. *Quarterly Journal of Studies on Alcoho4 15*, 562-586.

Keeler, M. H., Taylor, C. I., & Miller, W. C. (1979). Are all recently detoxified alcoholics depressed? *American Journal of Psychiatry, 136*, 586-588.

Kernberg, 0. (1975). *Borderline conditions and pathological narcissism.* Northvale, NJ: Aronson.

Khantzian, E. J. (1985). The self-medication hypothesis of addictive disorders: Focus on heroin and cocaine dependence. *American Journal of Psychiatry, 142*, 1259-1263.

Kohut, H. (1971). *The Analysis of the Sell* Madison, CT: International Universities Press.

Kikbler-Ross, E. (1969). *On death and dying* New York: Macmillan. Leshner, A. I. (1996). Understanding drug addiction: Implications for treatment. *Hospital Practice, 31(10)*, 47-54,57-59.

Marsh, M., Cohen, M. E., & Tucker, M. B. (Eds.). (1982). *Women's use of drugs and alcohol: New perspectives.* New York: Plenum Press.

Martin, C. (1984). An historical review of Georgia's impaired physician's program. *Journal of the Medical Association of Georgia, 74*, 745-748.

Martin, C. A., & Talbott, G. D. (1986). Women physicians in the Georgia impaired physicians program. *Journal of the Medical Association of Georgia, 75,*483-488.

Martin, C. A., & Talbott, G. D. (1987). Special issues for female impaired physicians. *Journal of the American Medical Women's Association, 42,* 115-121.

McCrady, B., Longabaugh, R, Fink, E., Robert, S., Beattie, M., & Ruggierri-Authelet, A. (1986). Cost effectiveness of alcoholism treatment in partial hospital versus inpatient settings after brief inpatient treatment: 12-month outcomes. *Journal of Consulting and Clinical Psychology, 54,*708-713.

Meisch, R. (1991). Studies of drug self-administration. *Psychiatric Annals, 21,* 230-234.

Miller, N., & Chappel, J. (1991). History of the disease concept. *Psychiatric Annals, 21,* 196-205.

Miller, N., Dackis, D., & Gold, M. (1987). The relationship of addiction, tolerance, and dependence to alcohol and drugs: A neurochemical approach. *Journal of Substance Abuse Treatment, 4,* 197-207.

Miller, N. S., & Hoffmann, N. G. (1995). Addictions treatment outcomes: Special issue — Treatment of the addictions: Applications of outcomes, research for clinical management. *Alcoholism Treatment Quarterly, 12(2),* 41-55.

Mirin, S., Weiss, R., Michael, J., & Griffin, M. (1988). Psychopathology in substance abusers: Diagnosis and treatment. *American Journal of Drug and Alcohol Abuse, 14,* 139-157.

Morrison, M. (1989). *White rabbit.* New York: Berkley.

Morse, R., & Flavin, D. (1992). The definition of alcoholism. *Journal of the American Medical Association, 268,* 1012-1014.

Morse, R., Martin, M., Swenson, W., & Niven, R. (1984). Prognosis of physicians treated for alcoholism and drug dependence. *Journal of the American Medical Association, 251,* 743-746.

Noble, E. (1991). Genetic studies of alcoholism: CNS functioning and molecular biology. *Psychiatry Annals, 21,* 215-229.

O'Malley, S. S.Jaffe, A. J., Chang, G., Schottenfield, R. S., Meyer, R. E., & Rounsaville, B. (1992). Naltrexone and coping skills therapy for alcohol dependence: A controlled study. *Archives of General Psychiatry, 49,* 881-887.

Porter, T., & Smoot, S. (1996). A description of patients treated from 1975-1996: Talbott Recovery Systems, Atlanta, Georgia. (Unpublished manuscript)

Porter, T., Talbott, G. D., & Irons, R. (1994). Addiction treatment outcomes: A seven-year follow-up study. (Unpublished manuscript)

Reading, E. (1992). Nine years experience with chemically dependent physicians: The New Jersey experience. *Maryland Medical Journal, 41,* 325-329.

Reuler, J., Girard, D., & Cooney, T. (1985). Wernicke's encephalopathy. *New England Journal of Medicine, 312,* 1035-1039.

Robinowitz, C. B. (1983). *The physician as a patient.* In S. C. Scheiber & B. B. Doyle (Eds.), *The impaired physician.* New York: Plenum Medical.

Rose, K. B., & Rosow, I. L. (1972). Marital stability among physicians. *California Medicine, 16,* 95-99.

Rosenthal, M. (1984). Therapeutic communities: A treatment alternative for many but not *all. Journal of Substance Abuse Treatment, 1,* 55-58.

Rounsaville, B. J., Beissman, M. M., Crits-Christoph, K., Wilber, C., & Kleber, H. (1982). Diagnosis and symptoms of depression in opiate addicts: Course and relationship to treatment outcome. *Archives of General Psychiatry, 39,* 151-156.

Rounsaville, B. J., Rosenberger, P., Wilber, C., Weissman, M. M., & Kleber, H. D. (1980). A comparison of the SADS/RDC and the DSM-III. *Journal of Nervous and Mental Disease, 168,* 9097.

Sargeant, J. K., Bruce, M. L., Florio, L. P., & Weissman, N. M. (1990). Factors associated with one-year outcome of major depression in the community. *Archives of General Psychiatry, 47*(6), 519-526.

Satir, V. (1988). *The new peoplemaking.* Mountain View, CA: Science & Behavior.

Savitz, S., & Kolodner, G. (1977). Day hospital treatment of alcoholism. *Current Psychiatric Therapies, 17,* 257-263.

Schaef, A. W. (1986). *Codependence misunderstood – Mistreated.* Minneapolis: Winston Press.

Schuckit, M. (1981). Twin studies on substance abuse: An overview.

Progress in Clinical and Biological Research, 69 (Pt. C), 61-70. Schuckit, M. A. (1983). Alcoholism and other psychiatric disor-

ders. *Hospital and Community Psychiatry,* 4,1022-1027.

Schuckit, M. A. (1985). Genetics and the risk of alcoholism. Journal *of the American Medical Association, 254,* 2614-2617.

Schuckit, M. A. (1986). Genetic and clinical implications of alcoholism and affective disorder. *American Journal of Psychiatry, 143,* 140-147.

Shore, J. (1987). The Oregon experience with impaired physicians on probation: An eight-year follow-up. *Journal of the American Medical Association, 25Z* 2931-2934.

Smith, P. C., & Smith, J. D. (1991). Treatment outcomes of impaired physicians in Oklahoma. *Journal of the Oklahoma State Medical Association, 84,* 599-603.

Snow, C., & Willard, D. (1989). *I'm dying to take care of you.* Redmond, WA: Professional Counselor.

Subby, R. (1990). *Healing the family within.* Deerfield Beach, FL: Health Communications.

Talbott, G. D. (1982). The impaired physician and intervention: A key to recovery. *Journal of the Florida Medical Association, 69,* 793-797.

Talbott, G. (1984). Elements of the impaired physician program.

Journal of the Medical Association of Georgia, 73, 749-751. Talbott, G. D., & Cooney, M. (1982). *Today's disease: Alcohol and drug dependence.* Springfield, IL: Charles C. Thomas.

Talbott, G. D., & Gallegos, K. V. (1990). Intervention with health professionals. *Addiction and Recovery, 10(3)*, 13-16.

Talbott, G. D., Gallegos, K. V., Wilson, P., & Porter, T. L. (1987). The medical association of Georgia's impaired physicians program— Review of the first 1,000 physicians: Analysis of specialty. *Journal of the American Medical Association, 257*, 2927-2930.

Talbott, G. D., & Gander, 0. (1975). Alcoholism the disease: A medical fact. *Journal of the Medical Association of Georgia, 64*, 331-333.

Talbott, G. D., Holderfield, H., Shoemaker, K. E., & Atkins, E. C. (1976). The Disabled Doctors Plan for Georgia. *Journal of the Medical Association of Georgia, 65*, 71-76.

Talbott, G. D., & Martin, C. (1984). Relapse and recovery: Special issues for chemically dependent physicians. *Journal of the Medical Association of Georgia, 73*, 763-769.

Talbott, G. D., & Martin, C. A. (1986). Treating impaired physi-

cians: Fourteen keys to success. *Virginia Medical, 113*, 95-99. Talbott, G. D., & Porter, T. (1994). The relapsing physician when

short-term treatment fails. (Unpublished manuscript)

Tarasoff v. Regents of the University of California. (1974). 118 Cal. Rptr. 129, 529 P.2d 553: on reh'g (1976), 17 Cal. 3d 425, 551 P.2d 334, 131 Cal. Rptr. 14.

Tarter, R. E., Hegedus, A. M., Goldstein, G., Shelly, C., & Alterman, A. I. (1984). Adolescent sons of alcoholics: Neuropsychological and personality characteristics. *Alcoholism, Clinical & Experimental Research, 8*, 216-222.

Tesch, B. J., Wood, H. M., Helwig, H. L., & Butler-Nattinger, A. B. (1995). Promotion of women physicians in academic medicine—Glass ceiling or sticky floor, *Journal of the American Medical Association, 273(13)*, pp. 1022-1025.

Tiverski, A. J. (1982). *It happens to doctors, too.* Center City, MN: Hazelden.

Vaillant, G. E. (1970). Physicians' use of mood altering drugs: A 20-year follow-up report. *New England Journal of Medicine, 272,* 365-370.

Vaillant, G. E. (1980). The doctor's dilemma. In G. Edwards & M. Grant (Eds.), *Alcoholism treatment in transition* (pp. 37-59). Baltimore: University Park Press.

Vaillant, G. E. (1983). *The natural course of alcoholism.* Cambridge, MA. Harvard University Press.

Vaillant, G. E. (1996). A long-term follow-up of male alcohol abuse. *Archives of General Psychiatry, 53,* 243-249.

Vaillant, G. E., Sobowale, N. C., & McArthur, C. (1972). Some psychological vulnerabilities of physicians. *New England Journal of Medicine, 287,* 372-375.

Vincent, M. 0. (1976). Female physicians as psychiatric patients. *Canadian Psychiatric Association Journal, 1,* 461-465.

Wallace, J. (1977). Alcoholism from the inside out: A phenomenological analysis. In N. J. Estes & M. E. Heinemann (Eds.), *Alcoholism: Development, consequences, and interaction* (pp. 110-115). St. Louis: C. V. Mosby.

Webster, T. G. (1983). Problems of drug addiction and alcoholism among physicians. In S. C. Scheiber & B. Boyle (Eds.), *The impaired physician* (pp. 97-103). New York: Plenum.

Wegscheider-Cruse, S. (1990). *Understanding codependency.* Deerfield Beach, FL: Health Communications.

Weiss, R., & Mirin, S. (1985). Treatment of chronic cocaine abuse and attention deficit disorder, residual type with magnesium pemoline. *Journal of Drug and Alcohol Dependence, 15,* 69-72.

Weissman, M. M., & Myers, J. K. (1980). Clinical depression in alcoholism. *American Journal of Psychiatry, 137,* 372-373.

Wise, R. (1987). The role of reward pathways in the development of drug dependence. *Pharmacology and Therapeutics, 35,* 227-263.

REFERENCES

Woodruff, R. A., Jr., Guze, S. B., Clayton, P. J., & Carr, D. (1973). Alcoholism and depression. *Archives of General Psychiatry, 28(1)*, 97-100.

Woolf, D. S., & Bennett, G. (1983). Health professionals in substance abuse treatment. In G. Bennett, C. Vourakis, & D. S. Woolf (Eds.), *Substance abuse: Pharmacological, development, and clinical perspectives* (pp. 428-434). New York: Wiley.

Zuska, J. J., & Pursch, J. A. (1980). Long-term management. In S. E. Gitlow & H. S. Peyster (Eds.), *Alcoholism: A practical treatment guide* (pp. 131-163). New York: Grune & Stratton.

Appendix

For further information regarding physician health issues and individual state physician health programs, please contact:

Federation of State Physician Health Programs
1430 Main Street
Waltham, MA 02154
1-800-322-2303 or (781) 893-4610

President
John A. Fromson, M.D.
Massachusetts Medical Society, Physician Health Services
President-Elect
Lynn Hankes, M.D.
Washington Physicians Health Program
Immediate Past-President
Gerald L. Sumner, M.D.
The Medical Association of the State of Alabama, Physicians
Recovery Network
Secretary
Linda Kuhn
Texas Medical Association, Committee on Physician Health
and Rehabilitation Treasurer
William M. Moclair, RN
Rhode Island Medical Society, Physicians Health Committee

Author Index

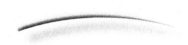

Subject Index

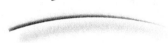

CPSIA information can be obtained at www.ICGtesting.com
Printed in the USA
BVOW08s1710090215

386983BV00010B/73/P